The Authorities

Powerful Wisdom from Leaders in the Field

DR. STEVE OH
Stem Cell Scientist and Entrepreneur

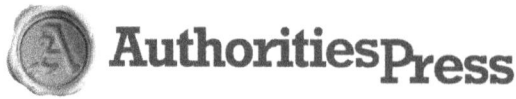

Copyright © 2017 Authorities Press

ISBN-13: 978-1977973672
ISBN-10: 1977973671

All rights reserved. No portion of this book may be reproduced mechanically, electronically, or by any other means, including photocopying, without permission of the publisher or author except in the case of brief quotations embodied in critical articles and reviews. It is illegal to copy this book, post it to a website, or distribute it by any other means without permission from the publisher or author.

Limits of Liability and Disclaimer of Warranty

The author and publisher shall not be liable for your misuse of the enclosed material. This book is strictly for informational and educational purposes.

Warning – Disclaimer

The purpose of this book is to educate and entertain. The author and/or publisher do not guarantee that anyone following these techniques, suggestions, tips, ideas, or strategies will become successful. The author and/or publisher shall have neither liability nor responsibility to anyone with respect to any loss or damage caused, or alleged to be caused, directly or indirectly by the information contained in this book.

Medical Disclaimer

The medical or health information in this book is provided as an information resource only, and is not to be used or relied on for any diagnostic or treatment purposes. This information is not intended to be patient education, does not create any patient-physician relationship, and should not be used as a substitute for professional diagnosis and treatment.

Publisher
Authorities Press
Markham, ON
Canada

Printed in the United States, Canada and United Kingdom.

FOREWORD

Experts are to be admired for their knowledge, but they often remain unrecognized by the general public because they save their information and insights for paying customers and clients. There are many experts in a given field, but their impact is limited to the handful of people with whom they work.

Unlike experts, authorities share their knowledge and expertise far more broadly, so they make a big impact on the world. Authorities become known and admired as leading experts and, as such, typically do very well economically and professionally. Most authorities are also mature enough to know that part of the joy of monetary success is the accompanying moral and spiritual obligation to give back.

Many people want to learn and work with well-respected and generous authorities, but don't always know where to find them. They may be known to their peers, or within a specific community, but have not had the opportunity to reach a wider audience. At one time, they might have submitted a proposal to the For Dummies or Chicken Soup for the Soul series of books, but it's now almost impossible to get accepted as a new author in such branded book series.

It is more than fitting that Raymond Aaron, an internationally known and respected authority in his own right, would be the one to recognize the need for a new venue in which authorities could share their considerable knowledge with readers everywhere. As the only author ever to be included in both of the book series mentioned above, Raymond has had the opportunity to give back and he understands how crucial it is for authorities to have a platform from which to share their expertise.

I have known and worked with Raymond for a number of years and consider him a valued friend and talented coach. He knows how to spot talented and knowledgeable people and he desires to see them prosper. Over the years, success coaching and speaking engagements around the world have made it possible for Raymond to meet many of these talented authorities. He recognizes and relates to their passion and enthusiasm for what they do, as well as their desire to share what they know. He tells me that's why he created this new nonfiction branded book series, The Authorities.

Dr. Nido Qubein
President, High Point University

TABLE OF CONTENTS

Introduction V

Personal Stem Cell Banking - To Increase Your LONGEVITY 1
Dr. Steve Oh

The 3 Things You Need to Become a Real Estate Millionaire 19
Raymond Aaron

Happiness: How to Experience the "Real Deals" 25
Marci Shimoff

Sex, Love and Relationships 35
Dr. John Gray

The Greatest Weapon Against Cancer Is Knowledge 41
Melanie R. Palomares, M.D., M.S.

One Step at a Time 59
Parents, Educators and Children with Autism share their success stories
Anne-Carol Sharples

Awakening Your Healer Within…The Miracle of You! 73
Philip Young

The Modern Healer 91
Herman Siu and Martin Siu

How To Gain Abundant Wealth 109
Kay Eve

The Secret to Words 129
Jacqueline Lucien

How to Make Your Advertisement Infinitely More Effective 141
Francis Ablola

Have More Money, More Clients and More Freedom
by Going Digital 159
Ashar Alam

INTRODUCTION

This book introduces you to *The Authorities* — individuals who have distinguished themselves in life and in business. Authorities make a big impact on the world. Authorities are leaders in their chosen fields. Authorities typically do very well financially, and are evolved enough to know that part of the joy of monetary success is the accompanying social, moral and spiritual obligation to give back.

Authorities are not just outstanding. They are also *known* to be outstanding.

This additional element begins to explain the difference between two strategic business and life concepts — one that seems great, but isn't, and the other that fills in the essential missing gap of the first.

The first concept is "the expert."

What is an expert? The real definition is …

EXPERT: *a person who knows stuff*

People who have attained a very senior academic degree (like a PhD or an MD) definitely know stuff. People who read voraciously and retain what they read definitely know stuff. Unfortunately, just because you know stuff does not mean that anyone respects the fact that you do. Even though some experts are successful, alas, most are not — because knowing stuff is not enough.

Well, then, what is the missing piece?

What the expert lacks, "the authority" has. The authority both knows stuff and is *known* to know stuff. So, more simply …

AUTHORITY: *a person who is known as an expert*

The difference is not subtle. The difference is not merely semantic. The difference is enormous.

When it comes to this subject, there are actually three categories in which people fall:

- People who don't know much and are unsuccessful in life and in business. Most people fall in this category.

- People who know stuff, but still don't leave much of a footprint in the world. There are a lot of people like this.

- Experts who are also *known* as experts become authorities and authorities are always wondrously successful. Authorities are able to contribute more to humanity through both their chosen work and their giving back.

Some of *The Authorities* in this book are world-famous. Others are just as exceptional, but you may not yet know about them. Take our featured author, Dr. Steve Oh, as an example. He is the Institute Scientist of the Stem Cell Group at the Bioprocessing Technology Institute (BTI), A*STAR (Agency for Science Technology and Research), in Singapore. His career has been dedicated to developing robust bioprocessing technologies for the manufacture of adult and pluripotent stem cells, with an irrepressible vision of seeing cell therapies succeed in the clinic and ultimately benefiting patients. Steve has been a Biotech professional for 27 years with experience at the National University of Singapore and the Fortune 500 company Pall Corporation. For 17 of those years, he has been in stem cell research. His vision is to bring large scale, personalised stem cell therapy to the world in partnership with companies and academics engaged in this multifaceted exercise. He's currently crafting the research programme at BTI to create the Future of Stem Cell Manufacturing as an industrial cluster. He has started 2 companies with his inventions and runs a research team of 20 staff members working in adult and pluripotent stem cells, as well as immunotherapy.

Serving on various committees of the International Society of Cellular Therapy (ISCT), Steve enjoys shaping policies to legislate cell-based treatments and is dedicated to growing the awareness and importance of cellular remedies through webinars, presentations and publications. His latest book, Sensational Stem Cells! How to cure medical complications, reduces the complexity of this field, plainly to the public. Steve is considered an authority in his field.

Read each chapter carefully to learn and to see the business potential that may be possible between yourself and each one of *The Authorities*. You may well be able to become their client or, possibly, do business with them in other ways.

They are *The Authorities*. Learn from them. Connect with them. Let them uplift you. Learning from them and working with them is the secret ingredient for success which may well allow you to rise to the level of Authority soon.

To be considered for inclusion in a subsequent edition of *The Authorities*, register to attend a future event at www.aaron.com/events where you will be interviewed and considered.

Personal Stem Cell Banking

To Increase Your LONGEVITY
DR. STEVE OH

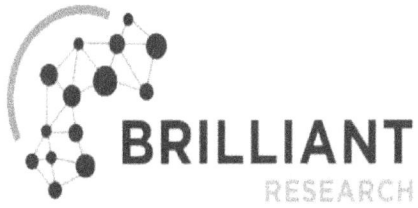

Our Vision

To be world leading stem cell pioneers, while also advancing the health of individuals.

Our Mission

Through dedicated research and development, we consistently provide best-in-class stem cell technologies.

Corporate Profile

The application of stem cells within therapy is a significant and thrilling advancement in healthcare, for research institutions and clinics alike. Coined as the Third Pillar in Healthcare, it will revolutionize the way medical professionals provide health solutions for patients. For research, an enriched understanding in molecular and physiological changes will increase medical professionals' understanding of disease development and therefore define new potential therapeutic strategies. For clinics, enhancing therapies through the application of stem cells has created the potential to regenerate and repair damaged tissue. Current therapies, such as bone marrow transplants, are already leveraging on this critical advancement. The challenge is therefore in the production of healthy stem cells to ensure the continued advancement of the healthcare sector.

Brilliant Research Pte. Ltd. ("Brilliant Research") endeavors to overcome these challenges head on by specializing in the development of stem cell research products, production tools and therapy products. In total, accomplishing these goals will ensure the continued evolution of the third pillar of the healthcare sector. Brilliant Research was founded on research from several leading-edge institutions, such as the Agency for Science, and Technology and Research (A*STAR), to ensure best-in-class quality products are delivered.

Brilliant Research was incorporated in response to the market demand for an increase in the number of stem cells for therapy in the production process and the ability to ensure each stem cell is healthy. Based in Singapore, Brilliant Research is able to leverage on a foundation of advanced research in a collaborative biomedical environment.

Brilliant Research believes not only in the advancement of health, which has been personalised to the individual, but also its people, products and services offered to customers and industry partners. By establishing sustainable relationships with employees, customers and partners, Brilliant Research is able to enhance its specialist capabilities so to better serve its customer base.

POTENTIAL OF STEM CELLS

Stem cells are remarkable due to their potential to develop into many different cell types in the body during early life and growth. Additionally, for many tissues they serve as a form of an internal repair system, which essentially divide without limit to replenish other cells during the period of a person or animal's life. When a stem cell divides, each new cell has the potential either to remain a stem cell or become another type of cell with a more specialized function, such as a muscle cell, a red blood cell, or a brain cell.

Stem cells are different from other cell types because of two important characteristics. The first reason is that they are unspecialized cells capable of renewing themselves through cell division. This sometimes happens even after long periods of inactivity. The second reason is under certain physiologic or experimental conditions they can be induced to become tissue- or organ-specific cells with special functions. In some organs, such as the gut and bone marrow, stem cells regularly divide to repair and replace worn out or damaged tissues. In other organs, however, such as the pancreas and the heart, stem cells only divide under special conditions.

Stem cell's unique regenerative abilities offer lots of new potential for treating diseases such as diabetes, and heart disease. However, there is still a lot of work that needs to be done in the laboratory and the clinic to understand how to use these cells for cell-based-therapies to treat disease.

Human stem cells have a variety of ways to be used in research and the clinic. Studies of human embryonic stem cells will be able to provide new information about the complex events that occur during human development. One of the primary goals of work on these cells is to identify how undifferentiated stem cells become the differentiated cells that form the tissues and organs. Scientists know that being able to turn genes on and off is central to this process. Some of the most serious medical conditions that the world faces today are due to abnormal cell division and differentiation. This includes diseases such as cancer and things like birth defects. As the scientific community gains more complete understanding of the genetic and molecular controls of these processes we should get information about how such diseases arise and develop new strategies for therapy. To be able to predictably control cell proliferation and differentiation further research into the molecular and genetic signals that regulate cell division and specialization will be required. While recent developments with induced pluripotent stem cells suggest some of the specific factors that may be involved, techniques must be devised to introduce these factors safely into the cells and control the processes that are induced by these factors.

Human stem cells are also currently involved in a new drug testing procedure. Differentiated cells generated from human pluripotent cell lines are now used to test the safety of new medications. There is a long history of using other kinds of cell lines in this way. An example of this is cancer cell lines which are used to screen potential anti-tumor drugs. The availability of pluripotent stem cells would allow drug testing in a wider range of cell types. However, in order to screen drugs effectively, the conditions must be identical when comparing different drugs. For this reason, scientists must first be able to precisely control the differentiation of stem cells into the specific cell type on which drugs will be tested. For some cell types and tissues, current knowledge of the signals controlling differentiation falls short of being able to mimic these conditions precisely. Therefore, currently we often lack the ability to generate pure populations of differentiated cells for each drug being tested.

What is likely to become one of the most important potential application of human stem cells is the generation of cells and tissues that could be used for cell based therapies. A common issue today is the need of donated organs and tissues, which are often used to replace ailing or destroyed tissue, far outweighs the available supply. Stem cells, directed to differentiate into specific cell types, offer the possibility of a renewable source of replacement cells and tissues to treat diseases including macular degeneration, spinal cord injury, stroke, burns, heart disease, diabetes, osteoarthritis, and rheumatoid arthritis.

Promising research shows that it may become possible to generate healthy heart muscle cells in the laboratory and then transplant those cells into patients with chronic heart disease. Through preliminary research it has been found that when bone marrow stromal cells are transplanted into a damaged heart of mice and other animals there can be beneficial effects. There are several reasons why these cells may help and scientists and health professionals are actively investigating these. It could be that they generate heart muscle cells or stimulate the growth of new blood vessels that repopulate the heart tissue, or help via some other mechanism. For example, injected cells may accomplish repair by secreting growth factors, rather than actually incorporating into the heart. Promising results from animal studies have served as the basis for a small number of exploratory studies in humans.

People who suffer from type 1 diabetes are victims of an autoimmune disease where their own immune system attacks and destroys the cells of the pancreas that normally produce insulin. New studies indicate that it may be possible to direct the differentiation of human embryonic stem cells in cell culture to form insulin-producing cells that eventually could be used in transplantation therapy for persons with diabetes.

To realize the promise of novel cell-based therapies for such pervasive and debilitating diseases, scientists must be able to manipulate stem cells so that they possess the necessary characteristics for successful differentiation, transplantation, and engraftment. The following is a list of steps in successful cell-based treatments that scientists will have to learn to control to bring such treatments to the clinic. To be useful for transplant purposes, stem cells must be reproducibly made to:

- Reprogrammed safely from human donor material to pluripotent stem cells.
- Proliferate extensively and generate sufficient quantities of cells for making tissue.
- Differentiate into the desired cell type(s).
- Survive in the recipient after transplant.
- Integrate into the surrounding tissue after transplant.
- Function appropriately for the duration of the recipient's life.
- Avoid harming the recipient in any way.

Also, to avoid the problem of immune rejection, scientists are experimenting with different research strategies to generate tissues that will not be rejected. To summarize, stem cells offer exciting promise for future therapies, but significant technical hurdles remain that will only be overcome through years of intensive research.

CURRENT STATE OF THE MARKET

International stem cell powers, well aware of the enormous potential of stem cell R&D, are moving quickly:

- Japan has committed more than $1 billion to accelerate clinical application of research using induced pluripotent stem cells.
- In the United States, California has committed more than $3 billion to stem cell research and regenerative medicine over 10 years. New York $550 million over 11 years. Maryland: $100 million over five years.
- The United Kingdom is investing heavily in regenerative medicine and its House of Lords recently recommended that Britain act now to prevent falling behind the U.S. and Japan.[1]

BCC Research projects that the global stem cell market will grow from about $5.6 billion in 2013 to nearly $10.6 billion in 2018, registering a compound annual growth rate (CAGR) of 13.6% from 2013 through 2018.[2]

The global stem cell bio banking market is estimated to be valued at USD 1.58 Billion in 2016 and projected to grow at a CAGR of 20.2% from 2016 to reach USD 3.96 Billion by 2021. The storage services sector holds the largest market share in the stem cell bio banking market. Increasing awareness regarding the storage of cord blood and tissue stem cells, high growth potential of emerging economies, and increasing use of stem cells in the field of therapeutics have opened an array of opportunities for the growth of the market in coming years.[3]

OPPORTUNITIES FOR INVESTORS

We are currently seeking strategic investments from Angel Investors or Venture Capital Funds for 2 business opportunities:

1. A Personalised Stem Cell Banking for high net worth individuals to bank their own stem cells for health insurance and future medical needs.

2. A Stem Cells Research Business which will provide novel tools for stem cell researchers globally.

These business themes are elaborated in more detail in the following pages.

PERSONALIZED STEM CELL BANKING FROM BLOOD CELLS

One of the most exciting breakthroughs driving personalized medicine today is stem cell therapy. Of particular promise is a specific type of therapy known as autologous stem cell treatments using personalized pluripotent stem cells. Brilliant Research offers personalized stem cell banking of pluripotent stem-cells made from a client's own blood so you are poised to take advantage of any medical or other breakthroughs using these high potential cells!

This sounds complicated at first but it's really quite simple at its core. Autologous therapy is the process where the stem cells used in a treatment come from a patient's own body while pluripotent stem cells are a particular type of stem cell which are proving to have the most versatile and powerful properties. Figure 1 on page 9 depicts the process that Brilliant Research will be offering. Blood from the donor will be transformed into human induced pluripotent stem cells using Brilliant Research's patented technology. These human induced pluripotent stem cells will then be banked in long term storage for future use, when cell therapies become common place within 5 years. They can be turned into heart, neural and blood cells as examples, for curing a wide range of medical ailments.

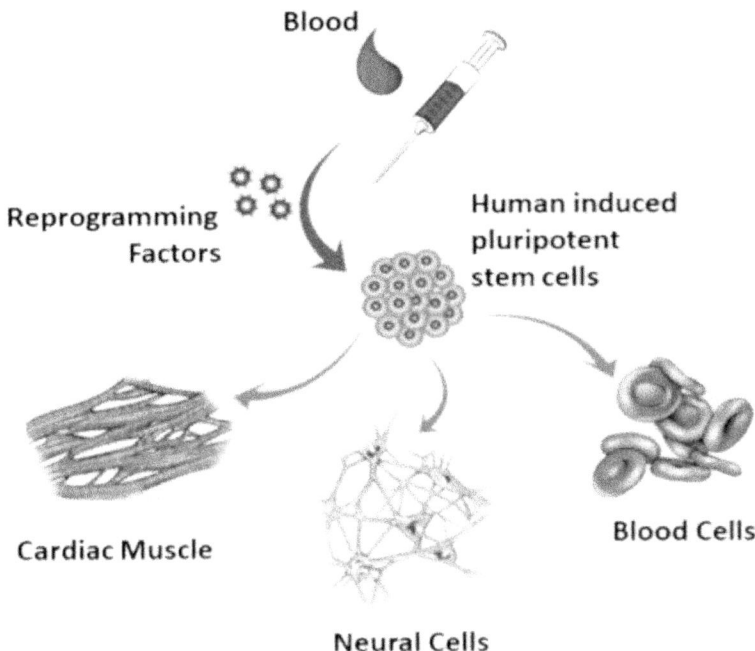

Figure 1. Reprogramming blood cells to induced pluripotent stem cells for personalised stem cell banking. These pluripotent stem cells can become any cell type in the body.

Many laboratory studies are beginning to show that stem cell treatments conducted using your own pluripotent stem cells can effectively halt, treat, and even in some cases reverse disease. What is truly remarkable about this is that these particular stem cells are not limited to develop into one cell type since they are pluripotent. This means they can give rise to any other cell type in the body, from blood cells, muscle cells, liver, islet cells to neural cells and bone cells.

This makes stem cell therapy a highly attractive alternative to current drug-based and physical therapy treatments, which tend to only temporarily manage symptoms.

Some of the benefits of pluripotent stem cell treatments over traditional methods include:

- Very low risk of immune rejection as seen in allogeneic stem cell treatments (when stem cells from a donor are used)
- No need to find a stem cell donor
- Minimal to no risk of needing anti-rejection drugs
- Very low risk of developing graft-versus-host disease (GVHD), a condition in which the transplanted donor stem cells attack the recipient's cells.
- Minimal risk of your body rejecting organ transplants

Cell-based treatments of this kind are just over the horizon. More importantly the technology and knowledge for extracting and storing your own pluripotent stem cells is already here. Not many laboratories or companies have the experience or skills to do this at a commercial scale yet. Brilliant Research is building the automation platform to do this!

While stem cells can be harvested from a patient at any age, the younger you are, the more versatile and healthier your stem cells are. As you age, your stem cells' regenerative ability will slow down. This is why preserving your stem cells early in life at an adult pluripotent stem cell bank is crucial. This will make sure there is no delay in getting the most modern treatments when they become available or when you are in the greatest need. By doing this as soon as you can, you are ensuring you are extracting your cells when you are still healthy and the youngest you will ever be.

These approaches to personalized medicine often utilize stem cells to accomplish these goals. However, stem cells can be negatively affected by donor variables such as age and health status at the time of collection, compromising their efficacy. The stem cell banking offered by Brilliant Research gives you the opportunity to cryogenically preserve stem cells at their most potent state for later use in these applications. However, this process is time consuming and expensive. Foresight now can and will save you a headache in the future. By storing your stem cells with us you are not only ensuring quick future access but guaranteeing their existence in an uncertain future. A situation can always arise where you may truly need them and at that time you are not guaranteed to be able to afford the cost to make them either monetarily available or useful time-wise.

Pluripotent stem cell derivatives provide a uniquely scalable source of functional differentiated cells that can potentially repair damaged or diseased tissues to treat a wide spectrum of diseases and injuries. Almost every day the media reports on the development of new stem cell breakthroughs and discoveries. There is no doubt that stem cells have the potential to treat many human afflictions, including cancer, diabetes, blindness, neurodegeneration and ageing. While some of these are still science fiction many are reaching towards clinical applicability. If a breakthrough happens you will need to already have stem cells on hand to take advantage of it quickly.

Please email Dr. Steve Oh at Brilliant Research - steve@brilliant-research.com or go to his website - www.brilliant-research.com

The following list describes areas where stem cell research funding is going and where progress toward cures is currently happening:

Research Stage (10-20 years to Therapy)

- Alzheimer's disease

- Amyotrophic lateral sclerosis (ALS or Lou Gehrig's disease)
- Arterial limb disease
- Arthritis
- Autism
- Cancer: Brain tumor
- Cancer: Leukemia
- Cancer: Skin
- Cancer: Solid tumor
- Deafness
- HIV/AIDS
- Huntington's disease
- Kidney disease
- Multiple sclerosis
- Respiratory disease
- SCID/Primary Immune Diseases
- Sickle cell disease

Clinical Stage (5-10 years to Therapy)
- Blindness
- Diabetes
- Heart disease
- Osteoporosis, bone and cartilage disease
- Parkinson's disease
- Spinal cord injury
- Stroke

STEM CELLS RESEARCH PLATFORM

Our patents, technologies and proprietary know-hows have been licensed from A*STAR which has several advanced institutions under its umbrella including the Bioprocessing Technology Institute (BTI), the Singapore BioImaging Consortium (SBIC), the Institute of Materials Research & Engineering (IMRE), and the Institute of Chemical Engineering Science (ICES). These combination of advancements and scientific discoveries has paved the way for the foundation of Brilliant Research products and service offerings.

The initial primary products available from Brilliant Research are patented stem cell research reagents and they are available in 3 broad categories:

Microcarriers – have been specially created for a) human pluripotent and b) adult human mesenchymal stem cell (hMSC) expansion and differentiation in both static culture plates and suspension spinner flasks or bioreactor cultures. The first line of products are designed for three broad applications: expansion of human embryonic stem cells (hESC) and human induced pluripotent stem cells (hiPSC); differentiation to embryoid bodies (EBs); directed differentiation to specific lineages for example – cardiomyocytes and neuroprogenitors. These microcarriers can be used in conventional plate cultures such as petri dishes, 6 and 12 well non-adherent plates, and in suspension cultures such as spinner/shake flasks and bioreactors. In the pipeline are microcarriers being developed for the expansion of hMSC in serum and serum free media in suspension cultures.

Labeling Agents – have been created for monitoring of hMSC. Live fluorescent probes/dyes have been developed for identifying stem cell proliferation or senescence.

Human Stem Cells – human pluripotent stem cells differentiated to cardiomyocytes and neuroprogenitors for research applications such as tissue engineering, toxicity assays or organoid development.

In addition to the patented stem cell reagents, Brilliant Research offers training in both theory and practical as well as consultancy services.[4]

Current services

- Bioprocess development scale-up and optimisation for stem cells.
- Serum free media development for suspension cultures.
- Integrated expansion and differentiation of pluripotent stem cells.
- Bioreactor fed batch cultures. Quality assessment and control of stem cells.
- Particulate assessment of the bioprocess.
- Purification of stem cells.
- Novel potency assay development.
- General education on stem cells basics.
- General education on stem cell therapies and clinical trials.
- Biologics

CURRENT PRODUCT TYPES

SenezRed™

SenezRed™ can be used for identifying, staining and imaging senescent MSC cells from different sources. SenezRed™ is a membrane-permeable fluorescent probe which selectively stains live, senescent mesenchymal stem cells. SenezRed™-labeled cells can be visualized using fluorescent imaging.

Efficacy demonstrated on umbilical cord MSCs, bone marrow MSCs and adipose MSCs.

SenezRed™ is the only labeling agent available in the market for live staining of senescent MSCs.

Applications include:

1. Simple and rapid labeling protocol.

2. Enables selective labeling of primary senescent, less-potent mesenchymal stem cells without fixation.

3. Can be used to label live cells for fluorescent imaging.

4. Can be potentially used as a process analytical tool for stem cell bioprocesses, and to track MSC in migration assays, co-culture systems, cell-cell communications and tumor tropism studies.

5. As part of a standardized QC protocol.

This product is for research only.

IPS-Spheres™

IPS-Spheres™ microcarriers (MCs) provide a foundation for the scalable and robust production of human pluripotent stem cell (hPSCs)-derived functional cells in large numbers, by means of an integrated propagation and differentiation bioprocess in a defined environment. The MCs can be used for generating uniform EBs-like cell aggregates under agitation cultures and subsequently directly differentiated towards various lineages or functional cells (e.g. cardiomyocytes and neural progenitor cells). The advantages of this approach are: high cell yields; scalable; controlled aggregate size; negligible labor-intensive manual intervention allowing expansion and differentiation of hPSCs in one vessel unit.

Applications include:

- Enables high cell yields for hPSCs expansion
- Can be used for directed differentiation to any lineages or functional cells with different medium, such as cardiomyocytes and neuroprogenitors
- Alternative to EBs formation, giving higher cell yields and easier handling than "cutting colonies" or Aggrewells
- This product is for research use only and is not for use in diagnostic procedures

MSC Production Kits (With MSC-Spheres)

All-in-one starter kit. This is a brand-new product launched by Brilliant Research which is able to produce 50 to 100 million MSC in a single disposable 100ml spinner flask culture on MSC-Spheres and allows easy harvesting of cells from the microcarriers. In addition, a vial of SenezRed dye is included for QC assay in this kit.

HESC-Derived Cardiomyocytes

Human cardiomyocytes differentiated from pluripotent stem cells are being used extensively in place of animal derived or donor harvested cardiomyocytes. They provide a more consistent and stable source of cells from established cell lines that have been used extensively in research labs. Brilliant Research now provides cardiomyocytes made with Genea Biocells' human embryonic stem cell line, GN19. By applying microcarrier technology, we can generate 100s of million to billions of cardiomyocytes for toxicology testing and tissue engineering and transplantation applications without researchers having to worry about producing the cardiomyocytes themselves. Brilliant Research can provide quantities ranging from 2 million to 100 million cells at competitive prices because of the very high yields generated by our proprietary technology. Cells can be delivered as a monolayer on microtiter plates or as cell microcarrier aggregates and transported at room temperate for easier shipping and replated on arrival. Larger quantities of 1 billion cells or more, can be custom produced. This product is for research purposes only.

Contact Prof. Steve Oh at Brilliant Research using the following email: steve@brilliant-research.com

Email Dr. Steve Oh at Brilliant Research - steve@brilliant-research.com or go to his website - www.brilliant-research.com

---

[1] (http://webarchive.nationalarchives.gov.uk/20130124071628/http://www.dh.gov.uk/prod_consum_dh/groups/dh_digitalassets/@dh/@en/documents/digitalasset/dh_4124088.pdf)

[2] (https://www.bccresearch.com/market-research/biotechnology/stem-cells-bio035e.html)

[3] (http://www.marketsandmarkets.com/Market-Reports/stem-cell-banking-market-220680183.html?gclid=Cj0KEQjwioHIBRCes6nP56Ti1IsBEiQAxxb5GxW3D4X5upXbovqee5T6n-1Ot5Ht1-_5Sxs0CzotsH8aAism8P8HAQ)

[4] (https://brilliant-research.com/solutions-service/contract-assay-services/)

The 3 Things You Need to Become a Real Estate Millionaire

The Right Way to Invest Successfully

RAYMOND AARON

It seems like everywhere you look, someone is claiming that they became a millionaire by investing in real estate, and encouraging you to do the same. There are lots of TV shows about flipping houses for a fast buck that make it appear as if it's easy to find the right property and just as easy to sell it in a matter of months for a good profit. Unfortunately, that's not really how it works.

Investing in real estate is a proven way to make money, a lot of it. You could end up with millions, but you could also make a lot of very costly mistakes along the way. There has been so much hype about how easy it is to become a real estate millionaire that many people jump into the market without knowing what they are doing, and that's a shame, especially because qualified help is available.

Anyone can invest successfully in real estate if they have three things: a great real estate mentor, a proven real estate system, and a way to correctly predict the future. In other words, you need someone smart and knowledgeable to guide you, an understanding of the financial and legal aspects of buying, holding and selling real estate, and an ability to see societal trends and visualize how those trends will impact the real estate market.

A GREAT REAL ESTATE MENTOR

Investing on your own can be financially dangerous, especially for a first-timer. You're dealing with a lot of money, so any mistake can be a huge one. Buying at the wrong time in the cycle can kill your investments. And, regardless of the real estate strategy you employ, you're bound to hold onto properties for some period of time which means that severe negative cash flow and vacancies can ruin you. Plus, bad property management and a failure to know the most recent real estate and tax laws can get you sued.

An experienced mentor can help you choose the best real estate strategies for your situation, and the right properties in which to invest. They can also help you avoid the many possible pitfalls and make money while holding properties, and counsel you on when to sell for a great profit. Working with the right mentor can also keep real estate investing from becoming your full-time job.

Many people find that some part of the investment process is uncomfortable for them, whether it's initiating a conversation with a realtor, submitting an offer or hiring a property manager. A mentor can be very helpful in such situations as well.

In sum, learning from and working with the right mentor can make you a highly profitable investor in a relatively short period of time. Look for someone with years of experience and a proven track record.

A PROVEN SYSTEM

There's much more to investing in real estate than "buy low, sell high." To be successful, you must have the correct facts and the correct monthly habits concerning your real estate. Overall, you need to know what to buy, when to buy it, whether there will be a positive cash flow while you're holding on to it, and when to sell. Plus, what is the right low? What is the right high? How much money do you have to put down and how much income must be generated while you're waiting to sell?

Determining if a property is a good buy takes a lot of research and analysis. You will need to look at comparable purchase prices in the area, as well as rental fees. You'll also need to consider the location, the age and condition of the building, tax rates and about 30 other pieces of data. Evaluating the information for just one property could take you a day or more.

If you're serious about becoming a real estate investor, you are going to be considering quite a lot of properties on a regular basis. Even if you want to make investing your day job, you'll never have the time necessary to research fully and evaluate every property that comes to your attention. Hence, the first part of your system has to involve weeding out the lesser opportunities and focusing on the ones with potential.

The investors I mentor learn how to determine if a property is really a great deal in seconds. You only need two pieces of data: the purchase price and the current rent rate. Compare the two using a two-part formula. First, divide the asking price (outgoing funds) by 100. Then, given that current mortgage interest rates are below 8-10% divide the number you got by two. If the current monthly rent doesn't meet or better that second number, eliminate the property from consideration.

As an example, say the asking price is $1 million. If you divide it by 100, it comes out to $10 thousand. Divide again, by two, and you get $5 thousand. If the monthly rent isn't $5 thousand or more, you should pass on the property. You may miss out on a few winners using this system but, if you eliminate more properties than you think you should, you'll be successful and safe. Remember that, if interest rates rise significantly, you will need to adjust the formula to compensate.

Once you've weeded out the chaff from the wheat, do your due diligence on the remaining properties. Work closely with your mentor during this part of the process and, again, when it comes to making deals, say no more than you say yes. Just don't get cold feet or shy away from a great deal.

In terms of timing, it all comes down to momentum. There is always an overall upward momentum. Real estate prices go up and down, on an upwards track. So, one good profit strategy is to buy low, watch values rise and sell during the next boom. More precisely, you want to buy just as prices rise off the bottom (so that they're already rising) and sell when prices hit double the bottom, which is typically the very minimum prices rise to at the peak of the ensuing boom.

Don't attempt to predict the extremes — you will make a significant amount of money more safely buying just after prices begin rising (not the lowest point) and selling towards the end of the up period —without the risk associated with waiting too long and missing the highest point.

You'll also need a system for monitoring your investments while holding on until it's time to sell. Having a strong property manager is essential. So is reviewing rents taken in versus uncollectibles, repairs, and other expenses to ensure that your cash flow remains positive.

PREDICTING THE FUTURE

Good real estate investors learn to identify marketplace trends and buyers' or renters' needs. Start by investigating and tracking growth trends by neighborhood: are prices rising, is an area getting ready for a renaissance, are there new job opportunities nearby or is the area close to another neighborhood that's gotten too pricey?

Great real estate investors, however, go far beyond those basics. They look for large demographic or social elements that might provide the next big opportunity. The huge number of returning veterans after World War II led to a Baby Boom that provides the perfect example. Every stage of their lives brought an opportunity for marketers, real estate builders, and other manufacturers to fill unmet needs, be it starter homes for when they had children, tricycles for those children who were too young to ride a bike, or new sizes and types of cars. All of this was predictable, but no one noticed. Opportunities were capitalized upon as they arose, but imagine what financial success could have been attained if someone had predicted the Baby Boomers' needs in advance.

And, now, those Boomers are driving the growth of retirement communities and nursing homes. But, they are a more independent lot than their parents were, and have strived to remain young and healthy as long as possible. Quite a few of them can still live and thrive on their own, but many may need a little help at this point in their lives. They don't need or want an aide, nurse or social worker on a full-time basis and certainly aren't ready for a nursing home. That means there is a huge need for more up-to-date, internet-ready independent supportive living arrangements, of which there are too few. Investing in one now is bound to be a win.

Don't forget that those Baby Boomers had children of their own, and that created a mini baby boom. Think about the ways in which those children, now middle-aged adults, are different from their parents and what needs they might have, especially regarding real estate. You might also consider whether changes in the workforce, higher divorce rates and the economics of leaving home after college have implications for the real estate market as well. Keep your eyes and minds open!

If you would like to learn more about winning strategies for investing in real estate, please visit http://rarestmonthlymentor.com.

Happiness: How to Experience the "Real Deals"

MARCI SHIMOFF

I was 41 years old, stretched out on a lounge chair by my pool and reflecting on my life. I had achieved all that I thought I needed to be happy.

You see, when I was a child, I thought there would be five main things that would ensure that I'd be happy: a successful career helping people, a loving husband, a comfortable home, a great body, and a wonderful circle of friends. After years of study, hard work, and a few "lucky breaks," I finally had them all. (Okay, so my body didn't quite look like Halle Berry's—but four out of five isn't bad!) You think I'd have been on the top of the world.

But surprisingly I wasn't. I felt an emptiness inside that the outer successes of life couldn't fill. I was also afraid that if I lost any of those things, I might be miserable. Sadly, I knew I wasn't alone in feeling this way.

While happiness is the one thing we all truly want, so few people really experience the deep and lasting fulfillment that fills our soul. Why aren't we finding it?

Because, in the words of the old country western song, we're looking for happiness in "all the wrong places."

Looking around, I saw that the happiest people I knew weren't the most successful and famous. Some were married, some were single. Some had lots of money, and some didn't have a dime. Some of them even had health challenges. From where I stood, there seemed to be no rhyme or reason to what made people happy. The obvious question became: *Could a person actually be happy for no reason?*

I had to find out.

So I threw myself into the study of happiness. I interviewed scores of scientists, as well as 100 unconditionally happy people. (I call them the Happy 100.) I delved into the research from the burgeoning field of positive psychology, the study of the positive traits that enable people to enjoy meaningful, fulfilling, and happy lives.

What I found changed my life. To share this knowledge with others, I wrote a book called *Happy for No Reason: 7 Steps to Being Happy from the Inside Out*.

One day, as I sat down to compile my findings, all the pieces of the puzzle fell into place. I had a simple, but profound "a-ha"—there's a continuum of happiness:

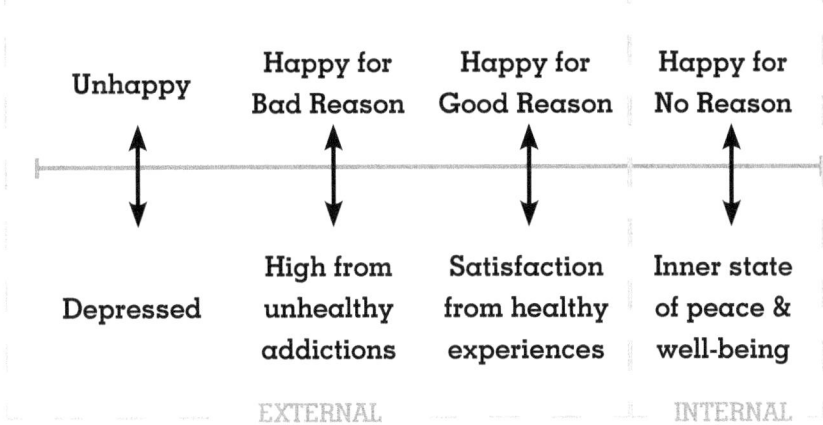

Unhappy: We all know what this means: life seems flat. Some of the signs are anxiety, fatigue, feeling blue or low—your "garden-variety" unhappiness. This isn't the same as clinical depression, which is characterized by deep despair and hopelessness that dramatically interferes with your ability to live a normal life, and for which professional help is absolutely necessary.

Happy for Bad Reason: When people are unhappy, they often try to make themselves feel better by indulging in addictions or behaviors that may feel good in the moment but are ultimately detrimental. They seek the highs that come from drugs, alcohol, excessive sex, "retail therapy," compulsive gambling, over-eating, and too much television-watching, to name a few. This kind of "happiness" is hardly happiness at all. It is only a temporary way to numb or escape our unhappiness through fleeting experiences of pleasure.

Happy for Good Reason: This is what people usually mean by happiness: having good relationships with our family and friends, success in our careers, financial security, a nice house or car, or using our talents and strengths well. It's the pleasure we derive from having the healthy things in our lives that we want.

Don't get me wrong. I'm all for this kind of happiness! It's just that it's only half the story. Being Happy for Good Reason depends on the external conditions of our lives—these conditions change or are lost, our happiness usually goes too. Relying solely on this type of happiness is where a lot of our fear is stemming from these days. We're afraid the things we think we need to be happy may be slipping from our grasp.

Deep inside, I think we all know that life isn't meant to be about getting by, numbing our pain, or having everything "under control." True happiness doesn't come from merely collecting an assortment of happy experiences. At our core, we know there's something more than this.

There is. It's the next level on the happiness continuum—Happy for No Reason.

Happy for No Reason: This is true happiness—a state of peace and well-being that isn't dependent on external circumstances.

Happy for No Reason isn't elation, euphoria, mood spikes, or peak experiences that don't last. It doesn't mean grinning like a fool 24/7 or experiencing a superficial high. Happy for No Reason isn't an emotion. In fact, when you are Happy for No Reason, you can have *any* emotion—including sadness, fear, anger or hurt—but you still experience that underlying state of peace and well-being.

When you're Happy for No Reason, you *bring* happiness to your outer experiences rather than trying to *extract* happiness from them. You don't need to manipulate the world around you to try to make yourself happy. You live from happiness, rather than *for* happiness.

This is a revolutionary concept. Most of us focus on being Happy for Good Reason, stringing together as many happy experiences as we can, like beads in a necklace, to create a happy life. We have to spend a lot of time and energy trying to find just the right beads so we can have a "happy necklace".

Being Happy for No Reason, in our necklace analogy, is like having a happy string. No matter what beads we put on our necklace—good, bad or indifferent—our inner experience, which is the string that runs through them all, is happy, and creates a happy life.

Happy for No Reason is a state that's been spoken of in virtually all spiritual and religious traditions throughout history. The concept is universal. In Buddhism, it is called causeless joy; in Christianity, the kingdom of Heaven within; and in Judaism it is called *ashrei*, an inner sense of holiness and health. In Islam it is called *falah*, happiness and well-being; and in Hinduism it is called *ananda*, or pure bliss. Some traditions refer to it as an enlightened or awakened state.

So how can you be Happy for No Reason?

Science is verifying the way. Researchers in the field of positive psychology have found that we each have a "happiness set-point," that determines our level of happiness. No matter what happens, whether it's something as exhilarating as winning the lottery or as challenging as a horrible accident, most people eventually return to their original happiness level. Like your weight set-point, which keeps the scale hovering around the same number, your happiness set-point will remain the same **unless you make a concerted effort to change it.** In the same way you'd crank up the thermostat to get comfortable on a chilly day, you actually have the power to reprogram your happiness set-point to a higher level of peace and well-being. The secret lies in practicing the habits of happiness.

Some books and programs will tell you that you can simply decide to be happy. They say just make up your mind to be happy—and you will be.

I don't agree.

You can't just decide to be happy, any more than you can decide to be fit or to be a great piano virtuoso and expect instant mastery. You can, however, decide to take the necessary steps, like exercising or taking piano lessons—and by practicing those skills, you can get in shape or give recitals. In the same way, you can become Happy for No Reason through practicing the habits of happy people.

All of your habitual thoughts and behaviors in the past have created specific neural pathways in the wiring in your brain, like grooves in a record. When we think or behave a certain way over and over, the neural pathway is strengthened and the groove becomes deeper—the way a well-traveled route through a field eventually becomes a clear-cut path. Unhappy people tend to have more negative neural pathways. This is why you can't just ignore the realities of your brain's wiring and *decide* to be happy! To raise your level of happiness, you have to create new grooves.

Scientists used to think that once a person reached adulthood, the brain was fairly well "set in stone" and there wasn't much you could do to change it. But new research is revealing exciting information about the brain's neuroplasticity: when you think, feel and act in different ways, the brain changes and actually rewires itself. You aren't doomed to the same negative neural pathways for your whole life. Leading brain researcher Dr. Richard Davidson, of the University of Wisconsin says, "Based on what we know of the plasticity of the brain, we can think of things like happiness and compassion as skills that are no different from learning to play a musical instrument or tennis …. it is possible to train our brains to be happy."

While a few of the Happy 100 I interviewed were born happy, most of them learned to be happy by practicing habits that supported their happiness. That means wherever you are on the happiness continuum, it's entirely in your power to raise your happiness level.

In the course of my research, I uncovered 21 core happiness habits that anyone can use to become happier and stay that way. You can find all 21 happiness habits at www.HappyForNoReason.com

Here are a few tips to get you started:

1. **Incline Your Mind Toward Joy.** Have you noticed that your mind tends to register the negative events in your life more than the positive? If you get ten compliments in a day and one criticism, what do you remember? For most people, it's the criticism. Scientists call this our "negativity bias" — our primitive survival wiring that causes us to pay more attention to the negative than the positive. To reverse this bias, get into the daily habit of consciously registering the positive around you: the sun on your skin, the taste of a favorite food, a smile or kind word from a co-worker or friend. Once you notice something positive, take a moment to savor it deeply and feel it; make it more than just a mental observation. Spend 20 seconds soaking up the happiness you feel.

2. **Let Love Lead.** One way to power up your heart's flow is by sending loving kindness to your friends and family, as well as strangers you pass on the street. Next time you're waiting for the elevator at work, stuck in a line at the store or caught up in traffic, send a silent wish to the people you see for their happiness, well-being, and health. Simply wishing others well switches on the "pump" in your own heart that generates love and creates a strong current of happiness.

3. **Lighten Your Load.** To make a habit of letting go of worries and negative thoughts, start by letting go on the physical level. Cultural anthropologist Angeles Arrien recommends giving or throwing away 27 items a day for nine days. This deceptively simple practice will help you break attachments that no longer serve you.

4. **Make Your Cells Happy.** Your brain contains a veritable pharmacopeia of natural happiness-enhancing neurochemicals — endorphins, serotonin, oxytocin, and dopamine — just waiting to be released to every organ and cell in your body. The way that you eat, move, rest, and even your facial expression can shift the balance of your body's feel-good-chemicals, or "Joy Juice", in your favor. To dispense some extra Joy Juice — smile. Scientists have discovered that smiling decreases stress hormones and boosts happiness chemicals, which increase the body's T-cells, reduce pain, and enhance relaxation. You may not feel like it, but smiling — even artificially to begin with — starts the ball rolling and will turn into a real smile in short order.

5. **Hang with the Happy.** We catch the emotions of those around us just like we catch their colds — it's called emotional contagion. So it's important to make wise choices about the company you keep. Create appropriate boundaries with emotional bullies and "happiness vampires" who suck the life out of you. Develop your happiness "dream team" — a mastermind or support group you meet with regularly to keep you steady on the path of raising your happiness.

"Happily ever after" isn't just for fairytales or for only the lucky few. Imagine experiencing inner peace and well-being as the backdrop for everything else in your life. When you're Happy for No Reason, it's not that your life always looks perfect — it's that, however it looks, you'll still be happy!

By Marci Shimoff. Based on the New York Times bestseller *Happy for No Reason: 7 Steps to Being Happy from the Inside Out*, which offers a revolutionary approach to experiencing deep and lasting happiness. The woman's face of the *Chicken Soup for the Soul* series and a featured teacher in *The Secret*, Marci is an authority on success, happiness, and the law of attraction. To order *Happy for No Reason* and receive free bonus gifts, go to www.happyfornoreason.com/mybook.

Sex, Love and Relationships

DR. JOHN GRAY

Just as great sex is important to lasting love, good health is important to sex and relationships. About 12 years ago, I cured myself of early stage Parkinson's disease. The doctors were amazed, but my wife was even more amazed. She noted that our relationship and sex life had become dramatically better. It turns out that the natural supplements I used to reverse Parkinson's can also make you more attentive and loving in your relationship. At that point, I realized that good relationship skills alone were not enough to sustain love and passion for a lifetime.

I shared many insights gained from my 40 years' experience as a marriage counselor and coach in *Men Are From Mars, Women Are From Venus*. And while my insights go a long way towards helping men and women understand and support each other, good communication skills alone are not always enough. For better relationships, we not only need to be healthy, but we must also experience optimum brain function.

If you are tired, depressed, anxious, not sleeping well, or in pain, then certainly romantic feelings will become a thing of the past. My recovery from Parkinson's revealed to me the profound connection between the quality of our health and our relationships. This insight has motivated me, over the past twelve years, to research the secrets of optimum health as a foundation for lasting love.

These are health secrets that are generally not explored in medical school. In medical school, doctors are indoctrinated into the culture of examining the symptoms, identifying the sickness, and prescribing a drug to treat that sickness. They learn very little about how to be healthy or to sustain successful relationships.

There are no university courses entitled "Better Nutrition For Better Sex". Drugs sometimes save lives, but they also have negative side effects that do little to preserve the passion in a relationship. Ideally, drugs should be used as a last resort and 90 % of our health plan should be drug free. From this perspective, the heath care crisis, as well as our high rate of divorce in America, is indirectly caused by our dependence on doctors and prescription drugs.

Most people have not even considered that taking prescribed drugs (even for the small stuff) can weaken their relationships, which in turn makes them more vulnerable to more disease. For example, if you are feeling depressed or anxious, a drug may numb your pain, but it does nothing to help you correct the cause of your problem. It can even prevent you from feeling your natural motivation to get the emotional support you need. In a variety of ways, our common health complaints are all expressions of two major conditions: our lack of education to identify and support unmet gender-specific emotional needs; and our lack of education to identify and support unmet gender-specific nutritional needs.

With an understanding of natural solutions that have been around for thousands of years, drugs are not needed to treat many common complaints. Some symptoms like low energy, weight gain, allergies, hormonal imbalance, mood swings, poor sleep, indigestion, lack of focus, ADD and ADHD, procrastination, low motivation, memory loss, decreased libido, PMS, vaginal dryness, muscle and joint pain, or the lack of passion in life and/or our relationships can be treated drug-free. By using drugs (even over-the-counter drugs) to treat these common complaints, our bodies and relationships are weakened, making us more vulnerable to bigger and more costly health challenges like cancer, diabetes, heart disease, auto-immune disease, dementia, and Alzheimer's. In simple terms, by handling the easy stuff (the common complaints) without doctors and drugs, we can protect ourselves from the big stuff (cancer, heart disease, dementia, etc.) We can be healthy and also enjoy lasting love and passion in our personal lives.

Even if you are taking anti-depressants or hormone replacement therapy, sometimes all it takes to stop treating the symptom is to directly handle the cause. With specific mineral orotates (something most people have never heard of) or omega three oil from the brains of salmon, your stress levels immediately drop and you begin to feel happy and in love again.

For every health challenge, we have explored the effects on our relationships, with as well as natural remedies that can sometimes produce immediate positive results. You can find these natural solutions to common health complaints for free at my website: www.MarsVenus.com.

What they don't teach in medical school is how to be healthy and happy without the use of drugs or hormone replacement. By refusing drugs and taking responsibility for your health, a wealth of new possibilities can become available to you. We are designed to be healthy and happy, and it is within our reach if we commit to increasing our knowledge.

New research regarding the brain differences in men and women reveals how specific nutritional supplements, combined with gender-specific relationship and self-nurturing skills, can stimulate the hormones of health, happiness and increased energy. Over the past 10 years in my healing center in California, I witnessed how natural solutions coupled with gender-specific relationship skills could solve our common health complaints without drugs. By addressing these common complaints without prescribed drugs, not only do we feel better, but our relationships have the potential to improve dramatically.

Ultimately the cause of all our common complaints is higher stress levels. Researchers around the world all agree that chronic stress levels in our bodies provide a basis for any and all disease to take hold. An easy and quick solution for lowering our stress reactions is specific nutritional support combined with gender-smart relationship skills. Extra nutritional support is needed because stress depletes the body very quickly of essential nutrients. When a car engine is running more quickly, it uses fuel more quickly. When we are stressed, we need both extra nutrients and extra emotional support. Understanding what we need to take and where to get it requires education. Every week day at www.MarsVenus.com I have a live daily show where I freely answer questions and provide this much-needed new gender-specific insight.

At www.MarsVenus.com, we are happy to share what we have learned for creating healthy bodies and positive relationships. You can find a host of natural solutions for common complaints and feel confident that you have the power to feel fully alive with an abundance of energy and positive feelings that will enrich all your relationships.

The Greatest Weapon Against Cancer Is Knowledge

Every Cancer Is Different. Learn About Your Risk And Ways To Reduce It

MELANIE R. PALOMARES, M.D., M.S.

Cancer afflicts millions of people and takes hundreds of thousands of lives each year. In 2012, the World Health Organization (WHO) reported 14 million new cancer diagnoses and 8.2 million deaths—and that number is projected to rise in the coming years.[1] Statistics suggest that about 39 percent of men and women will be diagnosed with this disease at some point during their lifetime.[2] The good news is that, today, early

---

1 World Health Organization Staff, "WHO | Cancer." World Health Organization, 2015. Web. http://www.who.int/mediacentre/factsheets/fs297/en/
2 National Cancer Institute Staff, "SEER Stat Fact Sheets: Cancer of Any Site." National Cancer Institute, 2013. Web. https://seer.cancer.gov/statfacts/html/all.html

detection and specialized treatment for different types of cancer can make all the difference.

Cancer used to be the disease that no one talked about—and, unfortunately, that meant that people at risk didn't even know about their family's medical history. Even today, there's a stigma surrounding cancer patients. In an article for *Cancer World*, the principal periodical of the European School of Oncology, Associate Editor Anna Wagstaff gives a harrowing report of the way societies around the world view cancer:

"Fears that the disease may be infectious can result in people being shunned by friends and neighbours (sic) and excluded from the community. Fears that it is hereditary can ruin the marriage chances of those with a mother or father known to have had cancer. Whole families can find themselves impacted, which can then put intolerable strains on relationships, leaving people with cancer even more isolated."[3]

The good news is that we are far more educated on the matter than we used to be. Today we have a wealth of information available via social media and the internet. The challenge is the quality of information available from such sources, which are not always subject to medical peer review. This has led to more awareness, and there have been more discoveries about lifestyle and environmental risk factors, which may be modified to improve cancer risk.

Studies have shown that the more accurate information one has, the better chance one has to maintain their health. In general, you are far more likely to survive a bout with cancer if you catch it at an early stage. For instance, Mayo Clinic reports the survival rate for colorectal cancer is 90% if it is caught early, although it is the second deadliest cancer in the United States, when all stages

---

[3] World Health Organization Staff, "WHO | Cancer." World Health Organization, 2015. Web. http://www. Anna Wagstaff, "Stigma: Breaking the Vicious Cycle." Cancer World, 2013. Web. http://www.cancerworld. org/Articles/Issues/55/July-August-2013/Patient-Voice/602/Stigma-breaking-the-vicious-cycle.html

are considered.[4]

This information may motivate you to pursue cancer screenings, but you should know that those come with their own set of risks. For one thing, screening tests are not 100% reliable. Even when they are conducted by medical professionals you know and trust, the possibility of a false-positive or false-negative result exists. Beyond that, some testing procedures come with their own immediate hazards. Colonoscopies, for example, carry some risk of damaging the lining of the colon.[5] Therefore, it is important to pursue to proper type and frequency of screening for your level of cancer risk.

By far, the best defenses against cancer are prevention and proactivity. The National Cancer Institute estimates that as many as 50-75% of cancer fatalities in the United States are caused by negative lifestyle choices, like smoking, lack of exercise, or poor diet.[6] Just by living a healthy lifestyle, you can reduce your chances of contracting cancer dramatically.

That said, it is most important to know how prone you are to the disease. If the disease runs in your family, or if you think that you may have had an exposure that may increase your risk of developing cancer (examples of such risk factors are discussed throughout this chapter), you need not feel helpless. Your first step is to talk with an oncologist or a general physician with specific training and experience in understanding cancer risk factors to perform an accurate risk assessment. From there, you can obtain personalized cancer screening recommendations tailored to your level of risk. You can also learn about a variety of different precautions that you can take to minimize

---

[4] Sharon Theimer, "Mayo Clinic Expert Shares Five Things to Know About Colorectal Cancer." Mayo Clinic News Network, 2016. Web. http://newsnetwork.mayoclinic.org/discussion/mayo-clinic-expert-shares-5-things-to-know-about-colorectal-cancer/
[5] National Cancer Institute, "Cancer Screening Overview." National Cancer Institute, 2016. Web. https://www.cancer.gov/about-cancer/screening/patient-screening-overview-pdq
[6] National Cancer Institute, NIH, DHHS. Cancer Trends Progress Report – 2011/2012 Update. Bethesda; 2012.

your chances of developing any form of cancer. It all comes down to having a keen knowledge of your personal history and knowing exactly what your body needs at any given time in your life, based on your age and occurrences in your life.

EVALUATING YOUR RISKS

When evaluating and minimizing your risk of developing cancer, it is important to note that one size does not fit all. Each form of cancer comes with a specific and distinct set of risk factors, variables that make you more or less susceptible to cancer development. In general, risk factors for cancer can be filed under two different classifications: genetic and environmental.

Genetic Risk Factors Are Inborn

Those with family histories of cancer, or those who inherit mutated genes from their parents, often have a relatively high chance of developing cancer. By nature, genetic risks are immutable and unalterable; we cannot, after all, change the way we were born. However, it is still important to recognize how your genes affect your chances of developing cancer, so that you may take appropriate preventive measures.

Environmental Risk Factors Are a Product of Nurture

These risk factors revolve around the characteristics of your living area, such as the climate (eg. sun exposure), the quality of the air you breathe, and the food you consume. Unlike genetic factors, environmental factors are, to some extent, subject to change. However, these changes may or may not be within your control, depending on what your living options are and whether you can afford to move.

In general, while there are many types and subtypes of cancer, all associated with different risk factors, screening, treatment, and prevention, in this chapter I will focus on the four most common cancers in the U.S.: breast and gynecologic cancers, colon cancer, lung cancer, and prostate cancer. These "Big Four" account for over 50% of all the cancers that occur in Americans.

BREAST AND GYNECOLOGIC CANCERS

From birth, sex hormones play an instrumental role in your body's growth, maturity and fertility. After you mature, your reproductive health is largely dependent on how well your body maintains the balance between estrogens and androgens. The enzyme aromatase plays a particularly vital part in a woman's reproductive health, breaking down larger hormones in the breasts and ovaries. This is important to note because breast cancer, like most gynecologic cancers, is hormone-driven.

The most important factors in determining breast cancer risk are gender and age. Since breast cancer growth is facilitated by the presence of female hormones, it serves to reason that the illness predominately affects women (but not only women). It also follows that breast cancer is most likely to develop post-maturity, when the body's hormonal activity reaches its peak. This is also the case for most ovarian and uterine cancers. On the other hand, cervical cancer is more likely to occur in young women, particularly those with more sexual activity, though the availability of human papilloma virus (HPV) vaccines will likely change the epidemiology of that disease as they become more commonly used for cancer prevention in girls and young women.

With breast and gynecologic cancers, despite popular belief, the role of inheritance is relatively minor. Although a family history of breast and/or ovarian cancer does make it more likely that you will develop one of these diseases, studies show that less than 15-20% of diagnosed breast cancer patients in America have immediate relatives with the same affliction,[7] and only about 5-10% have a strong family history of breast and/or ovarian cancer associated with a high cancer susceptibility genetic mutation. The most well-known examples are inherited mutations in the BRCA1 or BRCA2 genes, which are associated with the Hereditary Breast and Ovarian Cancer (HBOC) syndrome. Yet other cancer susceptibility genetic mutations, specifically mutations the DNA mismatch repair genes, are associated with a high risk of uterine and ovarian cancer with colon cancer, rather than breast cancer, in an entirely different inheritable entity called Lynch syndrome. In addition, there are gene mutations that carry only an intermediate elevation in risk for developing breast cancer, such as inherited mutations in a gene called PTEN, which are also associated with uterine cancer, thyroid cancer, and colon polyps as part of a less common familial entity called Cowden's syndrome. While there are even a few more familial syndromes that have been described to be associated with breast and/or gynecologic cancer, cervical cancer appears to be related to HPV infection as an environmental risk, with little to no relation to inheritance.

In addition to family history, you should also look into your personal history; breast cancer is more likely to happen in women who had their first period before age 12, as well as those who went through menopause relatively late.[8] The standard use of mammograms for breast cancer screening since the 1980s has shifted this disease to one that is more often caught early, except in younger women who may not have started regular screening yet. Two points

---

[7] breastcancer.org Staff, "U.S. Breast Cancer Statistics." breastcancer.org, 2016. Web. http://www.breastcancer.org/symptoms/understand_bc/statistics
[8] Mayo Clinic Staff, "Symptoms and Causes – Breast Cancer." Mayo Clinic, 2016. Web. http://www.mayoclinic.org/diseases-conditions/breast-cancer/symptoms-causes/dxc-20207918

follow from this trend: 1) women who have had findings of changes that occur prior to the development of a full cancer have an opportunity for medical prevention, and 2) it is particularly important to understand a woman's cancer risk in order to adjust screening recommendations to given high-risk women the same opportunity for early detection.

Lastly, diet and physical activity appear to play an important role in the development of these cancers. Obesity has been particularly associated with breast and uterine cancer. In addition, excessive alcohol use has been linked to breast cancer risk, particularly in premenopausal women.

COLORECTAL CANCERS

Colorectal cancers originate in the colon and rectum. The term "colorectal cancer" refers the most common of the cancers that develop within the human digestive tract. Colorectal cancers share a variety of causes and risk factors. One of them is chronic inflammation, as is seen in individuals with a history of the chronic inflammatory bowel diseases (IBD), Crohn's Disease or Ulcerative Colitis. Chronic inflammation can lead to the development of dysplasia, abnormally structured cells in the colon. Dysplastic cells often contain somatic, or non-inherited genetic mutations that are acquired after birth, which have the potential to develop into cancer cells over time.

Also, like breast and ovarian cancers, colorectal cancers have a familial component. In fact, there are some hereditary conditions that increase their carriers' propensity towards colorectal cancer. One such condition is Lynch syndrome, which was mentioned in the previous section, because of its association with uterine and ovarian cancers as well. Another syndrome is called familial adenomatous polyposis (FAP), an inherited condition that causes multiple polyps to grow in the patient's large intestine.[9] There are additional familial syndromes that have been described to be associated with colorectal cancers. These, as well as more detail about other cancer genetics syndromes, may be found at my website, www.caprevinc.org.

Diet is also thought to play a role in colon cancer, with certain elements, such as adequate folate and fiber intake, appearing to take an important role in minimizing risk.[10] Diets that include lots of vegetables, fruits, and whole grains have also been linked with a decreased risk of colon cancer. Dietary fat has been linked to a higher risk of colon cancer, as well as tobacco and alcohol use. The American Institute for Cancer Risk (AICR) estimates that 45% of colon cancers are preventable through diet, staying a healthy weight, and being physically active.[11]

LUNG CANCER

In general, lifestyle and environmental factors play the largest role in the development of lung cancer. This is an important point, in that lung cancer is the most common cause of cancer death in the United States, yet its risk factors are largely modifiable. Thus, it is important to understand these risks so that you can make the best choices for yourself and your family.

While tobacco use is the most well known risk factor, an additional major contributing factor is the exposure to secondhand smoke, or smoke expelled from used cigarettes and tobacco pipes. The American Cancer Society has

---

9 Al-Sukhni W, Aronson M, Gallinger S. "Hereditary colorectal cancer syndromes: familial adenomatous polyposis and lynch syndrome." Surg Clin North Am. 2008 Aug;88(4):819-44, vii. doi: 10.1016/j.suc.2008.04.012.

10 Giovannucci E, Willett WC. "Dietary factors and risk of colon cancer." Ann Med. 1994 Dec;26(6):443-52.

11 http://www.aicr.org/press/press-releases/preventing-colon-cancer-6-steps.html?referrer=https://www.google.com/

shown that secondhand smoke is even more toxic and carcinogenic than the vapor taken in by smokers themselves.[12] Because of this, the risk of lung cancer is relatively high for those who live or work around chronic smokers. Smoking and other tobacco use, such as chewing tobacco, also increases the risk for aerodigestive cancers, such as cancers of the oral cavity, throat, esophagus, and stomach. And because tobacco products can be excreted in the urine, tobacco use is also associated with kidney and bladder cancer.

Another large contributing factor to lung cancer is radon poisoning. Radon is a colorless, odorless substance that spawns from the natural decay of uranium in soil. Commonly, homes, particularly those in suburban or rural areas, can build up large quantities of radon over time as it rises up from the soil and seeps through cracks and flaws in the foundation. This is more common than you might think; in fact, it's responsible for roughly 21,000 lung cancer deaths each year, making it the second largest contributor to lung cancer behind tobacco.[13]

Asbestos is another major environmental factor associated with lung cancer. Asbestos poisoning is associated with a specific kind of lung cancer called mesothelioma. Since the 1980s, several laws have been passed in this country to restrict the availability and usage of asbestos in architecture. In spite of this, we still see a steady number of new mesothelioma diagnoses each year—about 3,000 annually, as estimated by the Mesothelioma Center.[14]

---

12 American Cancer Society, "Health Risks of Secondhand Smoke." ACS, 2015. Web. http://www.cancer.org/cancer/cancercauses/tobaccocancer/secondhand-smoke
13 Janet McCabe, "For peace of mind, add 'test for radon' to your 2016 to-do list." EPA Connect, 2016. Web.https://blog.epa.gov/blog/2016/01/test-for-radon/
14 The Mesothelioma Center, "Mesothelioma - Overview of Malignant Mesothelioma Cancer." asbestos.org, 2016. Web. https://www.asbestos.com/mesothelioma/

PROSTATE CANCER

Prostate cancer is the most common cancer occurring in American men, aside from skin cancer.[15] In 2016 alone, 26,120 American men were reported to have died from this affliction. In fact, one in seven men will be diagnosed with prostate cancer in their lifetime. Like breast and gynecologic cancers, prostate cancer is largely influenced by hormones; the difference, of course, is that it feeds off of androgens, male hormones, rather than estrogens.

Age is also a risk factor. Prostate cancer is seldom diagnosed in men younger than 40, and roughly 60% of cases are diagnosed in men at least 65 years of age.[16] Heredity and genes also play a role in prostate cancer development, although no highly penetrant cancer susceptibility genes have been described to date, unlike with breast, gynecologic, and colorectal cancers. Nevertheless, men who are closely related to prostate cancer patients are twice as likely to develop it themselves. The risk heightens even further if a man has more than one affected relative.

CANCER SCREENING

Cancer screening methods range from physical exam or self-exam to blood tests and specialized x-rays, such as mammograms, or procedures, such as colonoscopies. These methods are recommended to be performed at different frequencies depending upon age, family history, and other risk factors.

Concerns about false positive results, which can lead to unnecessary tests

---

15 Rebecca L. Siegel, Kimberly D. Miller and Ahmedin Jemal, "Cancer Statistics, 2016." CA: A Cancer Journal for Clinicians, 2016. Web. http://onlinelibrary.wiley.com/doi/10.3322/caac.21332/full
16 Prostate Cancer Foundation, "Prostate Cancer FAQs." Web. http://www.pcf.org/site/c.leJRIROrEpH/b.5800851/k.645A/Prostate_Cancer_FAQs.htm

and patient anxiety, as well as to overdiagnosis and overtreatment, has led to widespread controversy regarding different screening techniques. In addition, due to concerns about health care costs, cancer screening policies differ from country to country. This is why different guidelines are often offered by different medical organizations, which unfortunately leads to confusion for both consumers and health care professionals.

It is for this reason that I highly recommend seeking the advice of a physician with specific training and experience in understanding cancer risk factors to perform an accurate risk assessment. From there, you can obtain personalized recommendations specified to your risk level. Resources for determining your general category of cancer risk and, if appropriate, how to find a referral to a qualified health care professional near you can be found at my website, www.caprevinc.org. Webinars on this topic are in development and will be available at that site as well.

REDUCING YOUR RISK

While cancer screening can help with early detection of cancer, which does improve outcomes with cancer treatment, as mentioned earlier in this chapter, it is important to remember that you have the power to help mitigate your chances of developing cancer in the first place (or getting it again, if you are a cancer survivor). Fighting the disease is a matter of recognizing what you can and cannot control, and focusing on what you can control. Your personal choices on a day-to-day basis can make a huge difference in your personal war against cancer, and you cannot go into battle without knowing what the consequences of those choices are.

LIFESTYLE INTERVENTIONS

A balanced, careful diet is key to fighting cancer. The influence of your food intake on your cancer risk cannot be overstated. Some foods actually have the potential to increase your risk of developing cancer, so it's vital to know what to eat, what to abstain from, and what to limit.

Diet: Plant-Based Foods

When it comes to prevention of and survivorship with cancer, fruits, vegetables and whole grains are the most desirable foods you can eat. Cancer.net educates patients about the link between excessive body fat and the development of several types of cancer, including the aforementioned colorectal cancer.[17] As such, your best bet is to eat foods that are low in fat and high in fiber. Plant-based food groups (vegetables, fruits, nuts, whole grains and legumes) all fit the bill. Fiber-rich foods in particular will help you along the way. Fiber is the broom of the digestive system, sweeping your intestines clean and keeping your digestive processes running at regular intervals. Because of this, fiber helps flush carcinogenic compounds out of your body, thus preventing cancer from growing.

Diet: Animal Products

While a plant-based diet is wholly important to cancer prevention, this does not mean you have to swear off meat and dairy altogether. You should, however, place significant limits on how much animal-based food you take in. Most people, especially Americans, consume far more meat than they should.

---

[17] Cancer.net Editorial Board, "Obesity, Weight and Cancer Risk." Cancer.net, 2016. Web. http://www.cancer.net/navigating-cancer-care/prevention-and-healthy-living/obesity-and-cancer/obesity-weight-and-cancer-risk

In general, meat should not constitute more than a small fraction of the calories you take in per day. It's also important to recognize that some meats are better than others. Poultry and fish, for instance, are leaner and healthier alternatives to beef and pork. It's also a good idea to stay away from processed meats, like hot dogs and salami.

Physical Activity

Get moving! Exercise, particularly aerobic exercise, is an integral part of weight management, and by extension, cancer prevention. It is possible to reduce your risk for colorectal and breast cancer in particular with a regular exercise regimen. The AICR recommends sustained physical activity for at least 30 minutes a day.[18]

In addition to avoidance of obesity, which has been linked to an increasing number of different cancer types,[19] there are other benefits provided by regular exercise. For one thing, it keeps your metabolism running quickly and efficiently, which in turn will keep your weight at a healthy level. It also serves to strengthen your immune system, which plays an integral role in your body's defenses against cancer. Finally, regular exercise helps regulate your hormone levels which, as mentioned before, play a key role in the development of gynecologic cancers.

Stress Management

---

18 American Institute for Cancer Research, "Physical Activity Recommended for Preventing Cancer." AICR, 2016. Web. http://www.aicr.org/reduce-your-cancer-risk/recommendations-for-cancer-prevention/recommendations_02_activity.html

19 Béatrice Lauby-Secretan, Ph.D., Chiara Scoccianti, Ph.D., Dana Loomis, Ph.D., Yann Grosse, Ph.D., Franca Bianchini, Ph.D., and Kurt Straif, M.P.H., M.D., Ph.D., for the International Agency for Research on Cancer Handbook Working Group. Body Fatness and Cancer — Viewpoint of the IARC Working Group. N Engl J Med 2016; 375:794-798, August 25, 2016.

Chronic stress can affect body system functioning, particularly the immune system, and a weak immune system makes the body a more hospitable environment for cancer cells to grow. Stress also leads to release of a hormone called cortisol, which leads to truncal obesity, thereby leading to an increased risk of obesity-related cancers. Cortisol, along with other stress-related chemicals called catecholamines, has also been shown to directly facilitate cancer growth. Yet other stress hormones can inhibit a process called anoikis, which normally kills diseased cells and prevents them from spreading. Finally, chronic stress leads to increased production of growth factors that promote inflammation and new blood supply, which could potentially feed a developing cancer, as well as provide an environment for invasion and metastasis, or spread.[20]

While it is not realistic to avoid all sources of stress in our lives, it is possible to manage our relationship to external stressors. Mindfulness practices, such as meditation and yoga, can be very helpful in this regard. Getting adequate sleep not only supports successful stress management, but also allows to body to get the rest it needs to function well. Reading personal development books can help define knowledge and skills on how to manage situations that may be new or uncomfortable to us. Seeking the support of a mental health professional can be very helpful in identifying healthy ways to manage stress specific to your situation.

MEDICATIONS

If you are particularly worried about your susceptibility to cancer, there are a variety of cancer-suppressing medications that you can use. While some of them can be particularly potent cancer deterrents, they can be dangerous if

---

[20] Myrthala Moreno-Smith, Susan K Lutgendorf, and Anil K Sood, Impact of stress on cancer metastasis. Future Oncol. 2010 Dec; 6(12): 1863–1881.

used improperly. As with any drug, consult your physician before taking any of these medications, and be sure that you know about all of the side effects and potential risks.

For those with family histories of colon cancer, the Food and Drug Administration (FDA) recommends Celecoxib, most often known under the brand name 'Celebrex.' It works by disrupting the formation of polyps in your digestive tract, thus preventing cancer cells from growing there. However, those with histories of heart problems should be wary of using Celebrex. It is classified as a Non-Steroidal Anti-Inflammatory Drug (NSAID), and some NSAIDs can heighten your risk of heart disease and stroke.[21] In some patients, it may also cause serious gastrointestinal problems, including stomach ulcers.[22] Some studies suggest that aspirin may be an alternative for colon cancer risk reduction.

For breast cancer, there is a class of drugs known as selective estrogen response modifiers, or SERMs for short. In general, they have two primary functions; firstly, they are designed to suppress the production of estrogen in certain body tissues, particularly those in the breast. Secondly, they take on the functions that estrogen would normally fulfill, thus enabling your body to function properly without facilitating breast cancer growth.

But, like NSAIDs, SERMs have their own set of risks. Tamoxifen, for instance, heightens your risk of developing blood clots and having a stroke (though this risk is still relatively small). Tamoxifen can also exacerbate the symptoms of menopause, including hot flashes and vaginal dryness.[23] Tamoxifen has been shown to slightly increase the risk of uterine cancer, but for women who have a high risk for developing breast cancer, this risk is

---

21 The Internet Drug Index, "Celebrex." RxList, 2011. Web. http://www.rxlist.com/celebrex-drug.htm
22 Omudhome Ogbru, "Celebrex Side Effects Center." RxList, 2016. Web. http://www.rxlist.com/celebrex-side-effects-drug-center.htm
23 National Cancer Institute, "Hormone Therapy for Breast Cancer." 2012. Web. http://www.cancer.gov/cancertopics/factsheet/Therapy/hormone-therapy-breast

outweighed by its breast cancer reduction effects.

For postmenopausal women, an aromatase inhibitor called exemestane (brand name: Aromasin) is another alternative for medical breast cancer risk reduction. This drug may also be associated with menopausal symptoms, and also is associated with bone loss and thus may not be a good option for women with osteoporosis or osteopenia.

Prostate cancer patients have their own class of hormonal suppressant preventive agents, called 5α-reductase inhibitors. Two medications fall into this class of drugs, finasteride (brand name: Proscar) and dutasteride (Avodart). Similar to SERMs, they work by suppressing the production of androgens in the patient's body, thus preventing a cancer from growing. But, just like SERMS, these drugs may come with side effects.

Despite their side effects, these medications can be very useful for individuals with a high risk for a specific cancer, which underscores the importance of talking with your doctor about cancer risk assessment. If you are found to be at high risk, a cancer prevention specialist may offer you consultation to see if the benefits of a particular drug far outweigh its side effects in your particular case.

SURGICAL INTERVENTION

Preventive surgery is a last resort, as it can be stressful, risky and exceedingly expensive. It should only be used if your risk of developing cancer is high enough to justify it.

The most common form of preventive surgery is a bilateral mastectomy, the removal of one or both of your breasts. A mastectomy is often used to remove cancerous tissue in the breast, but it can also be used proactively to prevent the growth of cancer in that area. While a mastectomy will reduce the risk of breast cancer by a huge margin, it will not eliminate the risk altogether. Also, as you would expect, there are a variety of unrelated risks that come with the mastectomy procedure. Like any surgery, a mastectomy can lead to scarring, disfigurement, infection in the surgical area and blood clots. As such, only patients with an exceedingly high susceptibility to breast cancer should consider this option.

Similarly, prophylactic bilateral salpingo-oophorectomy (removal of both fallopian tubes and ovaries to prevent ovarian cancer) or prophylactic colectomy (removal of all or part of the colon to prevent colon cancer) may be considered in special high-risk patients.

These are just a few of the methods you can use to snuff out cancer before it grows. In short, the best way to minimize your chance of developing cancer is to take care of yourself. Have a keen awareness of what your body needs on a day-to-day basis, and act accordingly. Watch what you eat, keep track of your physical activity, and consult an experienced physician. If you'd like to learn more about the various types of cancer and what you can do to lower your own risk, please visit www.caprevinc.org or call 844-PREV-INC.

In summary, reducing your risk of getting cancer is possible. Start by understanding your family medical history as well as lifestyle and environmental risk factors. Have a positive attitude, a strict sense of self-awareness, and the willingness to change what you can and accept what you can't but with a proactive plan to manage your risk.

If you would like to know more about Dr. Melanie R. Palomares, M.D., M.S., and Cancer Prevention, Inc. please visit http://www.caprevinc.org/.

One Step at a Time

Parents, Educators and Children with Autism share their success stories

ANNE-CAROL SHARPLES

We all have aspirations and dreams for our children. Sometimes these expectations begin during our own childhoods as we dream about becoming parents. Sometimes the hopes and dreams do not begin until we look into the eyes of our newborn. No matter when the dream begins, no one dreams of autism. The diagnosis is a sucker-punch that leaves parents reeling and confused. Life quickly becomes complicated with all kinds of well-meant advice from professionals, family and strangers which include everything from medication to diet to the latest new therapy. This chapter does not offer advice on medicines, diet or therapies. The intention of this chapter is to uplift and inspire you. Perhaps you lay awake at night wondering, how I can fight the stigma related to the diagnosis. Maybe you cry, not because of who your child is, but because your child will not fit into the mold society expects. Please sit back and take a moment to learn about the successes of these autistic children and adults. It is with much love and respect that this chapter is dedicated to people on the autism spectrum as well as their families, teachers and caregivers.

SASHA

Sasha met all of her developmental milestones up until 22 months of age. It was then that the gregarious toddler fell silent. The daughter who was stringing two words together saying "What's this?" with inquisitive eyes vanished. Games and activities that Sasha once enjoyed no longer interested her. Eye contact became fleeting and she rarely responded to her name anymore. Sensing red flags, Sasha's parents Marjorie and Ryan began piecing the puzzle together. Shortly after, Sasha was diagnosed with autism. Devastated, but determined to bring back the vivacious child they once knew, the family began a courageous journey that would challenge every aspect of their personal relationships.

Investigating therapies, spending what seemed like hours on the phone and placing Sasha on waitlists left them disconcerted and worn out. Turning to one another for support, they drew upon each other's strengths and continued to map out the next steps in the journey. Together they discussed therapy options, and often reached for the other's hand when either one awoke panic stricken in the middle of the night, worried if they were doing the right thing.

Engaging Sasha in experiences and pulling her out of her shell that she so often retreated into became their undertaking. Sasha began Intensive Behavioral Intervention Therapy (IBI) on a daily basis. Family outings and activities took place every weekend. Rather than shielding Sasha from the world that overwhelmed her, her family wanted her to experience it in positive ways.

Sasha continued IBI until she turned four. It was then that Marjorie and Ryan registered her at the neighborhood school. Beginning kindergarten proved to be very challenging for Sasha and her family. The one-to-one therapy she'd been receiving each weekday was a stark contrast to the room filled with twenty-five boisterous children. IBI Therapy was usually quiet and controlled; the kindergarten classroom was anything but quiet! Sasha was overwhelmed and the first few weeks of school were traumatic for her. As Sasha entered the classroom each day a change would come over her. Her muscles tensed, arms and legs flailed, hands became fists and her jaw clamped shut. Sasha was in protective, fight mode. She was uncommunicative, confused and often distressed, making it impossible to participate in classroom activities. When the other children would sit in circle time and share their stories, she'd become increasingly agitated. Sasha's parents were quite concerned as she collapsed with exhaustion at the dinner table each evening, but they knew her adjustment would take time and vowed to continue taking her to school. What they did not know then, was that school would be the turning point for their daughter.

Marjorie and Ryan decided to use their beloved family outings as a way for Sasha to engage at school. They began to send in pictures of her with short anecdotes written on them. There were pictures of Sasha with her pet bird, at the pumpkin patch, visiting the zoo and opening presents on her birthday. On each of these pictures, Marjorie wrote about each day and what was occurring in the photograph. Over time, Sasha began to respond to these photos when her teacher shared them with her classmates during circle time. Slowly, with support from her teacher, Sasha began to sit for circle time. She'd become very excited when she saw a picture of herself. Sasha's teacher, Mrs. Watson, knew she wanted to share the stories of the pictures herself, so she would have Sasha stand beside her and share her stories through pointing and babbling. Sasha was beginning to communicate at school.

Mrs. Watson played a vital role in Sasha's success at school; for instance, she recognized that Sasha was overwhelmed by the large number of students in the class, so she assigned her a spot right next to her during circle time. She also introduced a visual schedule so that Sasha would know what to expect throughout her day. When there was an unanticipated disruption in her schedule, Mrs. Watson used an "Oops" card to demonstrate the change. Sasha began to communicate with Mrs. Watson by babbling and pointing to the pictures on her schedule. When she was hungry, she pointed to a picture of "snack." She even began to switch her schedule around to her preferred activities and would giggle while proudly showing Mrs. Watson the changes she had made. Sasha grew to love Mrs. Watson; she had a gentle tone of voice and made everyone feel welcome in her classroom. She made school fun for all of her students and her love for teaching shone through her interactions with the students. In addition to utilizing the photographs Sasha's parents sent in, she also recognized Sasha's love for books. Mrs. Watson provided her with a copy of the story she was reading to the class each day. Sasha could hold her book and look at the pictures while Mrs. Watson read aloud to the class. This was a simple yet effective way of keeping her engaged during story time.

Sasha was fortunate to have Mrs. Watson as her Senior Kindergarten teacher the following year. This is the year she began to speak. It began with a word mixed in with gibberish and pointing. It was easy enough to understand, so whoever Sasha was communicating with could model the appropriate language. Soon she began stringing two words together, then two became four so that "blah, blah backpack" became, "I want my backpack."

Sasha is now in first grade and loves school; she reads, writes and talks constantly. The other students adore Sasha because she is persistent, passionate and a joy to be around. She loves to share stories of family outings with her teachers and classmates, with or without photographs.

HENRY

When our son, Henry, was three years old, we were told that he'd never speak or be able to perform simple tasks. We watched, on pins and needles, as the developmental evaluator modeled the activity of stacking three blocks on top of each other and held our breath as she handed the blocks to Henry for him to duplicate what she'd done. Our hearts broke when he was unable to even attempt to stack them. After this evaluation, his father and I were told that Henry would need to be institutionalized. After the shedding of countless tears and multiple late night discussions, we knew that we would not put our son in an institution. We refused to give up hope that we could find a way to help Henry. We enrolled Henry in a school that offered special needs classrooms.

We were fortunate to find a wonderful group of teachers who worked tirelessly to see that Henry was able to function to the best of his ability. After two years in school, with the inclusion of daily therapy, he was able to communicate, albeit in a limited way. Henry never entered a mainstream classroom, but he has achieved multiple successes. The educators and assistants in Henry's special needs classrooms refused to accept the idea of can't. They repudiated the limitations that had been placed on Henry by various doctors and educational evaluators. They only saw what Henry could do and the sky was the limit as far as they were concerned.

Over the years Henry learned how to not only stack blocks, but to tie his shoes and dress himself. He will never hold a job or live by himself, but Henry has made huge strides from what we were originally told he would be able to accomplish. We know that institutionalization would not have been the best choice for Henry as he never would have progressed to the level that he is at today.

ABIGAIL

Here it was again, the dreaded block test. Abigail's grandmother, Eleanor, rolled her eyes as she watched the evaluator hand the blocks to Abigail. She knew Abigail would not stack the blocks or build the bridge the evaluator had shown her. Why are these blocks so important anyway she wondered? Abigail was four years old and had missed most of the developmental milestones. She was not yet speaking coherently; in fact, Abigail had little interest in speaking and seemed unconcerned if her needs were not met. She was absorbed by her own world and took little notice of anything occurring around her. Eleanor wondered if this was because Abigail's mother had abandoned her when she was eighteen months old. She suspected the troubles were compounded by issues in addition to abandonment and was not surprised by the diagnosis of autism. She was surprised when the healthcare professionals told her that Abigail would likely never speak or communicate because she was locked inside her own world. Institutionalization was mentioned, but quickly dismissed by Eleanor. She knew there was more for Abigail and held on to hope that she would find help for Abigail.

As it turned out, help was found during Abigail's first year of school. She started out at age five, a year behind most of the other children in the Junior Kindergarten class. Abigail's teachers and support staff read through the medical and behavioral evaluations and chose a course of action: Abigail was taught just as the other children were taught, with patience, love and repetition. Her teachers did not become frustrated when Abigail stared blankly and did not repeat the sounds they were asking her to make. Instead, they simply tried again the next day. Gradually, Abigail began to come out of her shell, appearing more aware and less self-absorbed. She haltingly began to repeat sounds, then words.

After two years of kindergarten, Abigail was speaking and able to communicate her needs and desires. Her comprehension moved more slowly; it was not until grade three that Abigail began to understand that she should take off her jacket when she felt warm. Her schoolwork moved slowly, as well. Her teachers spent extra time working with her each day and she worked with her grandmother and tutors in the afternoons and throughout summers.

Over the years, Abigail spent countless hours working after school with her tutors and teachers. Her grandmother worked tirelessly to see that Abigail reached her goals. Abigail graduated from high school and is now living on her own in an apartment with two other girls. She even has her dream job working at an amusement park she loved going to as a child.

MARIAH

My name is Mariah and I am twenty-one years old and I have autism. What autism means for me is that I am an excellent painter. I paint better than your average person does. I used to go to school, but now I am finished with school and can paint any time I want. This is very exciting for me because I love to paint; it's my favorite thing to do! My dad takes me and my paintings to art shows where we sell the paintings. My dad always says to do what you love and you will be happy.

MARIAH'S DAD

Mariah struggled with school. She is an excellent reader, but struggles with short-term memory and cannot recall recently taught basic math functions. She was teased often and never understood why the other kids didn't behave as she thought they should. She would often tell the other children what to do, an action that did not win her many friends. She didn't understand the rules of the playground and would push other kids off the swings when she wanted a turn. Her mother and I worried that she'd never be able to hold a job due to her lack of social skills and memory struggles. We wanted more for Mariah. We can provide for her financially, but wanted her life to have quality. We wanted Mariah to be joyful and content.

When she was in her first year of high school, Mariah took an art class and fell in love with painting. She loves the vivid colors and the feel of the paint. Her art teacher recognized that, not only did Mariah have a talent for painting, but that painting was restorative for Mariah. If Mariah was having a rough day at school, her teacher would bring her to the art room where she could calm herself with paint. Her mother and I were stunned at the artwork she brought home. Painting gives Mariah joy. She loves to go to art shows and speak with people about her paintings; she could talk about her paintings for hours! She has felt true success by giving enjoyment to others with her artwork. Since she is able to experience other people's reactions to her paintings, she is inspired to continue working on her craft. Mariah's struggles with interacting with other people evaporate when she speaks of her art. People may not understand Mariah's way of thinking, but they understand her art.

Art is the desire of a man to express himself, to record the reactions of his personality to the world he lives in. Amy Lowell, poet

LILY AND CHARLENE

Charlene will never forget the first day she met Lily. At that time, Lily's only way of communicating was to scream. Lily was four years old, an only child who lived in a low-income apartment with her father. At the time Charlene met her, Lily had received no prior intervention; she was a cautious girl who clung to her father's leg on that day in her apartment. While Lily's father was giving Charlene a snapshot of what the first four years of Lily's life had been like, Lily let it be known that she was displeased with the disruption to her routine. She screamed, climbed the furniture, and removed her clothing in protest. The volume of her screams pierced the air and her father worried that the neighbors would complain, yet again, about the noise. Her father explained that he had been unable to accomplish basics, such as getting Lily to sit in a chair to eat.

The years of struggle, both financial and emotional, wore on his face; he was desperate for help. His spirit was broken, beaten down by the everyday demands of life and compounded by his daughter's needs and his inability to understand her. Charlene desperately wanted to help and felt as though she were carrying a load of bricks as she walked away from their apartment, weighted down by the father's anguish for his daughter.

Charlene went to the school where she was employed as a support worker to speak with the principal about helping Lily. Principal Anderson's son is on the autism spectrum, so he related to the anguish Lily's father was experiencing. Plans were made and Lily began Junior Kindergarten the following week. To say that Lily's first day was exhausting for not only Lily, but also her dad and the staff would be an understatement. The five minute walk from their apartment building to the school took more than half an hour as Lily battled her father every step of the way. Upon arrival at school, it took another fifteen or so minutes for Lily's dad to convince her to enter the building. She made it to the threshold of the classroom and remained there all day long, screaming whenever anyone entered her space or tried to engage her. This continued for several weeks, and throughout that time Charlene persevered by remaining calm and respecting Lily's need for space. By doing this, Charlene gained Lily's trust along with the admiration of the classroom teacher and the staff within the school.

Charlene had a unique way of interacting with Lily; she understood that Lily's behavior was her only way of communicating. She treated Lily with dignity and respect and accepted her where she was. Charlene recognized how difficult school was for Lily and took baby-steps with her, acting as a guide who would remain with Lily until she was ready to go it alone. Over the weeks Lily moved from the threshold of the classroom door to learning how to sit inside the classroom, with Charlene at her side. This was accomplished with patience and kindness, but also with a song. "Row, Row, Row Your Boat" was sung to alert Lily that it was time to enter the classroom and sit down. Lily liked the song and began to request it by holding her hands out and rocking back and forth. Charlene found an old wooden boat and brought it into the classroom so that Lily could sit in the boat and rock it from side to side. This was a motivating experience for Lily since she loved to rock. It is from sitting in the boat that Lily learned how to sit in a chair.

Charlene shared the idea of singing the song with Lily's father. He began singing the song at home to alert Lily that it was time to sit down to eat. Her father was overjoyed when Lily joined him at the table, sat in a chair and shared a meal with him. Charlene was able to accomplish so much with Lily by taking the time to get to know and understand her. It is individuals like Charlene, who have an innate ability to be present and want to help, that make peoples' hearts smile. Lily's father's heart was smiling by the end of her Junior Kindergarten year as he found hope for his daughter's future.

CAITLIN

Mondays are the best. At least Caitlin thinks so because Monday is horseback riding day. Caitlin is fifteen years old and has been diagnosed with autism, in addition to several other health concerns. Caitlin does not have much energy and, as a general rule, does not enjoy exercise. However, she loves all things horse-related; she enthusiastically shows up for her horseback riding lesson and will brush her horse and clean out his stall with gusto. Not every day goes so well. Caitlin struggles when things do not go as she expects and some days Caitlin becomes irritated with her horse and kicks or even punches him out of frustration. Caitlin is working on developing patience, accommodating changes to routine and communicating with her horse without kicking or punching.

Her mother is thrilled with the life lessons, as well as the Hippotherapy Caitlin has received and has shared Caitlin's successes with her special needs classroom teacher, Mrs. McFray. Being quite perceptive, Mrs. McFray decided to explore Caitlin's interest in other animals. She learned that Caitlin has a passion for all animals; therefore, Mrs. McFray incorporated a classroom unit on animals and even obtained a grant to purchase several animals for her classroom. The animals, which include a turtle, a bunny, two guinea pigs and a hedgehog have been a huge hit with all of the students in the special needs classroom.

Caitlin's favorite is the bunny, Mr. Cuddles. She loves to feed him mint and watch him motor his way through the stalk. The students have learned that they cannot hold or pet an animal when they are angry because the animal will become frightened. Prickles, the hedgehog, rolls into a tight ball when she is scared or hears loud noises. Mrs. McFray believes that her students know exactly how Prickles feels. The students can only hold Prickles when they are quiet and calm; they are learning to self-regulate in order to interact with a classroom animal. The classroom pets are treasured by all; therefore the students are highly motivated to regulate their emotions. Because Mrs. McFray took the time to listen to Caitlin's mom, ponder what she heard, and explore options for incorporating animals in her classroom, all of the students have benefited. Mrs. McFray has a deep affection for her students and wants to offer each of them the best learning environment possible.

MILES

Hi, my name is Miles and I'm fourteen years old. I always knew there was something different about me, and it was confirmed when I was seven and told that I have Asperger's Syndrome. Fitting in at school, or anywhere else, has always been difficult for me. I wanted friends, but couldn't figure out how to make them. Things would start out okay, but after a while I noticed that my friends would not be around our usual hangouts. Even worse, when they'd see me they would turn their backs or walk away. I never understood what I'd done wrong. Having friends, then immediately losing them was the hardest part of school for me. The schoolwork was easy-peasy and I probably could've done it with my eyes closed. Recess was a nightmare. At least it was a nightmare until I met Mrs. Wiley and began attending the Program to Assist Social Thinking, aka PAST. I dedicate this story to her. It is due to Mrs. Wiley that I am where I am today.

I began attending PAST one day a week when I was in third grade and I liked it from the start. The best part of PAST is that it is a safe place where we can be ourselves and not worry about anything. You see, all of the kids who attend PAST have autism. And, all of the teachers are super cool and completely understand us. I feel comfortable in my own skin and I can be me when I'm there. Now, that doesn't mean that everything is fun and easy. My teachers challenge me all the time. They know exactly how far to push me and understand when I become frustrated. In fact, they taught me how to control my emotions. Mrs. Wiley, my parents, and my third grade teacher, Mrs. Smyth, would come up with goals I needed to work on at school and at home. So, one of the items my mom really wanted me to learn was how to ask her how her day was and to be genuinely interested in her response. One of the items my teacher wanted me to do was to greet her every morning. Each day I was rated on my performance and scores were tallied up weekly. Once I mastered these goals, other goals were set.

What makes PAST so much fun is that we do super-cool activities, like going rock climbing or to the aquarium that has sea life from around the world. Also, we have a Bearded Dragon in our class! In fact, Eragon, our Bearded Dragon, is such a popular guy, I don't think he is ever in his cage. He has a calming effect on all of us when we are upset. Another activity we do is sit on extremely cool bean bag chairs and do role plays. We also play games to learn about all sorts of barriers that prevent us from being social thinkers. One of my barriers is that I get stuck on what I want to do all of the time. At PAST we have to learn to work as a team and not just do what we want to do. We have a marble jar and each of us puts a marble in the jar when we are being social thinkers. Once the jar is full, we go on an outing; it could be eating at a neighborhood restaurant or checking out the largest indoor reptile zoo. We vote on it and decide. My teacher says we are working, but it feels more like fun than work!

I now realize that my friends used to avoid me as a result of me always wanting things my way. I wanted to be the boss of the whole shebang, from a game of soccer to only talking about what I wanted to talk about. Now I understand that it is important to let other people talk and to listen to them, even if I'm not all that interested. Mrs. Wiley and PAST have taught me how to interact with others and how to have a conversation. Now I know how to start and continue a conversation. PAST has taught me about the perspective of others. I used to think that everyone thought the same way I do. Well, I sure was surprised to find out this isn't so!

Anne Wiley retired from her role as a PAST Teacher in 2014 but continues to volunteer and contribute to the Autism Department at the TCDSB.

Awakening Your Healer Within

The Miracle of You!
PHILIP YOUNG

In this book you will glean information from "authorities" who offer mind-expanding ideas and concepts that will benefit your entire life and wellbeing. After countless hours of extensive study, thousands of client sessions, and twenty-five years experience, I am excited to be an authority. In my case, the particular subject of expertise is energetic healing and, like the other authorities in this book, I am pleased to share some of this information and knowledge with you. When learned and understood correctly, energetic healing has the ability to uplift, enlighten, and heal either you or a loved one.

To begin, we must define energetic healing. This is a metaphysical healing that takes place beyond the limits and assumptions of physical science known today. In reading this, you will learn how your inner, non-physical energy affects your health and wellbeing, and how this non-physical energy can be harnessed to assist you, sometimes in miraculous ways.

Today, most people see good health as something that is outside of their control, something that they have to fight to maintain. Health is also usually seen as that which is administered to them by outside medical experts and specialists, but there is another approach. What would it be like if, instead of seeking immediate traditional medical assistance, we embraced and recognized the body's own infinite wisdom? Could we then make changes from within? As people are able to open their minds to it, the answer to this question is most emphatically yes. All the wise and experienced physicians I've met with agree that, even with the scientific knowledge that has been gained over the years, we still know very, very little about the complexities of the human body. We are just beginning to scratch the surface of the miracle that we are.

The point of mentioning how little we know is to emphasize that there is another way of being, a way that truly 'does no harm' and is ultimately within your own control and power. If chosen, this is a path that leads to a radiant, healthier, and happier life that will help fill you with greater joy and wonder than ever before experienced.

Let's start with history. In ancient times it was understood that the natural state of human beings was one of vibrant health, and that this vibrant health came from the Self within. As science progressed, facts and data began to take precedence and this inherent knowledge was lost, buried, changed, or distorted. Now, millennia later, these truths are slowly being rediscovered.

I'd like to suggest that the secret of your entire health lies within you, and it is something that you can control with intention. It is something to be conscious of and to take responsibility for. This is a concept seldom taught or understood, which is especially regrettable because it takes so little commitment and discipline. In much the same way as other daily habits become routine, such as brushing your teeth, taking control of your health can be just that easy.

Many people regard themselves as victims or survivors of a disease (dis-ease), and this attitude has been encouraged in various ways in our society. It is a viewpoint that diminishes the Self and gives power to others. As you begin to consider yourself empowered as an active director of your own health, you engage your mind, spirit and body with intent, allowing miraculous changes to occur.

Every moment of every day, millions of cells are being created perfectly within your lungs, your organs, and your blood. All this takes place at the will of non-physical energy and is without any conscious effort on your part. It occurs simply by your inherent desire and intent. This is a monumental clue to the Truth and the beginning of realizing that you already are a miracle! This non-physical energy fills and actually enlivens your cells, tissues, and even your DNA. In fact, it permeates your entire being. Without being too esoteric, think of it as a 'Life Force', one that ultimately gives you Life and also determines your level of health and wellbeing. In circumstances when your health may not be currently optimal, this energy may have been compromised in some way. However, with help, application and some minimal training, it can be redirected to once again be a positive and beneficial resource for your body.

The dilemma that we have in our limited and often blinkered western way of looking at the world is that this non-physical energy has yet to be measured by material instruments. Society as a whole believes that, if something can't be measured, it cannot be. This line of reasoning actually mimics that of well-meaning priests from medieval times, who might have rigorously dismissed the concept of radio waves simply because they did not have the means to measure them at the time. That way of thinking is archaic. Non-physical energies can be perceived by those who are trained and considered to be attuned, open, and intuitively gifted. Moreover, the effects of these energies can be seen and experienced by all, whether or not we are aware of them.

For many years I have had the good fortune to help people experience healings that have been described as miraculous and even impossible. The people who have experienced healing have been able to reach a certain place within them of greater possibility. The process felt so natural, gentle, and effortless for them that they were often not even consciously aware of it taking place. In much the same way that you can use a magnifying glass to ignite kindling or paper, with my assistance people are able to reach a place of perfect health, a place Within that they ordinarily could not reach on their own.

So, how on earth do you reach the place Within that is already perfect? It is similar to tuning in to a radio station. In this case, however, you are tuning in to a subtle part of your Self. Continuing the radio metaphor, you may well experience some static, but if you persist you are able to tune in to that perfect part of you. As you invite the energy to come forth, hold a strong and consistent intent. Don't give up. When people struggle with this, occasionally they'll recall how they were when they were little children: carefree, happy, and hopefully in perfect health. A child's mind is filled with the exact joyfulness, openness and trust you are seeking. By holding onto these memories, the process may be easier.

To tune in to this station, it is also important to maintain a conscious feeling of gratitude for your perfect health in this very moment, regardless of present outward appearances. It's also important to suspend the activities of the intellect and ego and to control the mind chatter. You must move gently and in a state of deep relaxation through your feeling Self and through your loving Heart. By allowing yourself to maintain this thankfulness and gratitude for the miracle that you are, you can continue to fine tune this channel of perfection.

Because the process is unfamiliar, it can seem difficult at first. Most people find it far easier to begin with my help, and they always have beneficial results when they do. This occurs simply by my being fully Present with individuals in each visit with them. I speak with and listen to each person with patience and compassion. Using the vibration of my voice, and the heat and healing touch of my hands both on and around my clients' bodies, I'm able to help them find that place of perfection that's Within.

Over the years, I have found that there are always emotional hurts and concerns (real or imagined) that affect the wellbeing of the individual. Often, there are few if any people who have the time, patience, or compassion, and who are willing to listen to these concerns, much less respond in a supportive and loving way. Many doctors and specialists I meet sadly agree that they only have a few minutes to spend with each patient. Seldom do they learn much about the individual's hopes, past, fears, loves, concerns, personalities, relationships or families. So for them, if that were the case, it just wouldn't be possible to determine how non-physical energies may be of help to those in need.

When I meet clients in need of non-physical healing I allow the vibration of unconditional Love and highest intention to come forth. These energies can be felt as heat in my hands. Sometimes people actually think I have electric heating pads placed on their body. My own body becomes very warm, even hot, as these non-physical energies flow. It is a process of surrendering, of trusting without any ego whatsoever. Something much, much greater is present and in control. Usually this occurs for about an hour and then the energies stop, as the individual is complete. It is much the same way as we stop pouring water into a glass when it is full. No more can be added for the time being.

I feel most blessed to share these deep, sacred insights into the world of each individual. It allows for another aspect of their health, wellbeing and hope to blossom forth and then they feel better. True healing has to consider the totality of the person. It's a matter of body, mind, and spirit.

The following pages chronicle a few of the positive results I've obtained during my many years of practice. These anecdotal accounts demonstrate how real people have experienced wonderful results during healing sessions. Remember, if one man, woman, or child can do it, then so can another! Perhaps you are seeking a remedy at a time when other choices seem dim. If so, it could be that I might be able to help you or a loved one in some way. Whatever the reason, our Hearts and minds have crossed here for a sacred reason. I do hope that you enjoy the material on these pages and that you are inspired to implement the ideas for yourself, or perhaps to share them with others. Within the sanctity and authority of your own Self, take Heart, remain hopeful, and have faith that another way is surely at hand.

BREAST CANCER

"Your breasts are all clear."

Many years ago a dear and beloved friend called one day to say she had breast cancer. Little did I know then that her journey would help me embark on my own journey to becoming a healer.

Trish had been diagnosed with breast cancer and she was dreading the usual medical approach of "cut, poison, and burn" that still today seems to be the one size fits all medical standard. She had been endeavoring to learn as much as possible about her disease, including various alternative ways to treat her condition. She was fearful of chemotherapy's associated toxicity and the side effects that she knew would be so debilitating for her long-term health and wellness. She was open to another approach that was not harmful to her.

After many years of my own esoteric studies and interests, I was now faced with the stark reality of speaking my truth and endeavoring to do something for her or saying nothing while still trying to be supportive. Many of us have often found ourselves in similar situations. It's a matter of walking the talk vs. talking the talk.

I asked Trish if she was willing to try some healing after she had a lumpectomy. She answered yes and was, in fact, willing to try anything that might help. One day we sat down on her cottage lakefront and, to the bemusement of her husband and my wife, began to try a healing process I had read about. I felt certain and hopeful that I could really help her. That day, for about an hour we held the first of several such sessions, not really knowing what to expect, but highly desirous of a good outcome. Although these were just early steps at the time, nonetheless the good outcome arrived! Her breast cancer disappeared completely and to this day, over 20 years later, her breasts are cancer free!

LIFE SENTENCE

"We can't understand it. The tumors are gone."

Several months later I received a phone call from Jillian, a woman referred to me by Trish. Jillian had cancer throughout her body and had been diagnosed as only having a month or two to live. She was told to go home and get her affairs in order. We arranged to meet at her home and we spoke at length about what was going on in her life.

For the first five weeks we gently dealt with some personal issues that she had experienced. On each visit as I spoke with her I laid my hands upon her as she went into a deep guided relaxation. She returned to the hospital for follow up scans and tests, much to the amazement (and even anger, she said) of her medical doctors, as she had defied their diagnosis. Her tumors were either shrinking or had disappeared completely! Over the next several months she and I continued her healing sessions to the point where all tumors were completely gone.

I continued to see Jillian occasionally for over a two-year period. Years later, she eventually passed, but her life and vitality had been extended so much to the everlasting joy of her family, friends and loved ones.

COMA

"Your daughter is going to be in a permanent vegetative state. We are sorry, but there is no hope."

I happened to meet Rita by chance in an office where she was working. Rita told me her daughter Katrina had been struck by a car and had been thrown 70 feet. She had severe head trauma and had been in a coma for several weeks and, at this point, it was expected by the doctors that she would be in a permanent vegetative condition. There was nothing more they could do for her.

When I was a little boy I experienced head trauma and have always felt a deep sense of compassion and empathy for those who have head injuries.

When Rita told me about Katrina, I knew that I had to see her. Out of the blue, I asked Rita if she would be open to that and she said yes.

The next day, walking down the corridors of the hospital, part of me was asking what in the world I was doing there. Part of me wanted to get out of there before I made a complete fool of myself. And yet, another part of me was serene, sure, and calm. I felt like something was guiding me.

Rita was already in Katrina's room and we exchanged a few words. The doctors would not know what I'd be doing, but a couple of the nurses had been informed so that we would not be disturbed quite so much. Seeing Katrina so unresponsive on her bed was quite unsettling. What was I going to say to her? How could this possibly work without a verbal exchange? Without any feedback? With no clues from the eyes? Then I felt a still, calm knowing within me that became my guide. I moved the bed out from the wall, leaned over, and put my hands gently on first Katrina's head, then arm, then hand. Her mom simply looked on, accepting. After about 45 minutes, the healing session seemed to be complete. I really didn't know what to expect. This was new territory for me.

A day later, Rita phoned me to tell me that Katrina had moved her thumb and that the doctors had said this was a reflex. I replied that this is exactly the type of reflex we wanted! A few days later I went back to the hospital and repeated the session, gently touching her arm, her heart, as well as her head. Rita phoned again with good news; this time that Katrina had moved her arm. When I checked my messages a couple of days later I heard one from Rita. Katrina had spoken! I was so overjoyed to hear that and tears ran down my face. It was Christmas Day – what a gift! I saw Katrina several more times and I'm so thrilled that she made a full and quite miraculous recovery.

BRAIN BLOOD VESSEL PROBLEMS (AVM)

"I could drop dead at any moment."

Len was recommended by a friend after he was told by the medical specialists that he had a very serious malformation in the thalamus of his brain. The condition is called an arterio-venous malformation or AVM. There was a weakening in the walls of the blood vessels feeding this very intricate and important region of the brain and he was enduring terrible headaches and some numbness in his extremities. His doctors explained that the medical treatment for such a condition was gamma knife brain surgery. If he survived at all, he could have many cognitive deficits. If he did nothing, he left himself at risk of the malformation erupting and of inevitable sudden death. The odds were against him.

I was his last resort and our first meeting was brief. He was short on time and clearly short on inclination to believe in non-physical healing. He told me that he also had tendonitis from playing golf and wondered if I could do something for that, too. Before long he was soon on the massage table in a deep sleep-like state.

I thought things had gone well and after an hour brought him back. He said he felt unusually relaxed, yet he also seemed to be skeptical as to what he had just experienced. Not surprising for such a practical left brain thinking, alpha male. Still, he was very gracious and we said our farewells.

Sometimes, clients will call me soon after our sessions to let me know their good news. I hadn't heard from Len for several weeks and I was beginning to think that perhaps things had not gone so well for him, but then my phone rang. "Hi Philip, it's Len. I've been meaning to call you. The numbness in my extremities that I'd had for two years was gone the very next day after our session. Also, my stress was relieved and my tendonitis is completely gone too! Most importantly, I had another follow up MRI and the malformation has apparently shrunken from the size of a quarter to the size of a dime. The need for surgery has been averted."

The doctors apparently were astonished by the outcome. They said it was impossible.

Over the following year or two, I heard from Len asking for my assistance on a few other matters, including on behalf of a friend who had hurt her right shoulder ten years previously and could find no relief. She called me the very next day after that session. "I don't know what you did, but all the pain is now gone."

EPILEPSY

"I could black out at any time. I'll never drive or ride again."

Christine and I first met in a metaphysical/spiritual bookstore. We had lots in common and we became great friends. She is also into fitness and health, with a thriving home-based business on a ranch north of Toronto. In addition to caring for her animals, one of her greatest passions is driving a Harley Davidson. Recently, she had been experiencing epileptic seizures and was on strong medications to try and keep the unpredictable seizures under control. The prospect of no longer being able to drive or ride was a huge issue for her.

She was open to having some healing sessions, so I went to her ranch. Christine had three sessions, all of which went well. She now has a full and normal life, teaches yoga, and continues to ride her beloved Harley!

BLOCKED SALIVA GLAND

"I can't eat or drink. The pain is unbearable."

It was a bleak Monday evening in early December. The door opened slowly to reveal a tall, elegant young woman. I smiled and introduced myself and her eyes searched my face for a fleeting second, looking for…what? Hope, perhaps? With a wince of pain, she smiled back slightly.

We sat in her living room and, after exchanging pleasantries, she described her medical condition. Judy could not eat and could barely drink. On a pain and discomfort scale she was at a 10 plus. Her sub-mandible saliva gland duct was blocked with a large stone nearly 6mm (¼ inch) in size. The gland had also become infected. A prominent ENT (ear, nose, and throat) specialist had tried unsuccessfully in a two-hour operation to surgically remove the stone. She sought second opinions and all the ENTs had told her that the only medical recourse was to have her entire saliva gland removed. As a doctor herself she knew that a life without a saliva gland would also be intolerable, not to mention that there could also be permanent nerve damage to her face. She simply had to explore another avenue of possibility, no matter how outlandish it might seem, and thus the call to me.

Judy and I continued to speak at length about what was and had been going on in her life, recently and in the more distant past. A discomfort in her neck and jaw had been part of her life for nine years that seemed to worsen during emotional upset and stress. To me there was an obvious connection, but often the person suffering does not see it.

Judy seemed to be open to the possibility of non-physical healing, so after about 45 minutes we began. With some soothing music playing, I spoke quietly to her as she lay on my healing table. Slowly, she drifted away into a sleep-like state while I placed my hands gently on, around, and above her jaw, mouth, and neck. We ended our session and agreed to meet again in two days. I provided her with some positive thoughts and affirmations to focus on before our next session, that would allow the conscious and unconscious mind to do their parts to support the process further.

When we met again Judy's spirits seemed brighter and she was excited to report that the pain she had been experiencing had reduced significantly from a 10 to a more tolerable 4. She was no longer taking any Percocet for the pain.. During our talk, Judy said that her concerns were now more with the blockage and swelling under her tongue and the discharge from the infection. She rated both of these as a 9 out of 10 on the misery scale.

I reminded Judy of the miraculous being she was already and emphasized that in each and every moment her physical body was performing millions and millions of complex functions without any conscious effort on her part. Her Essential Self was taking care of all these functions. I suggested that this is a part of her that is not generally known to the conscious mind, the ego, or intellect. On the table once again, she drifted off into a relaxed sleep-like state while the energies flowed gently and lovingly in and around her being. As we completed, we again agreed to meet in two days time.

On my third visit Judy told me that after our last meeting she had run to the bathroom and had to spit something out. Amazingly, she was also able to eat again! Judy was excited to tell me that the misery index for the swelling under her tongue and the infection was now only at a 2! The pain had gone. There was only a small bubble under her tongue and only a very slight discomfort on the left side of her neck.

I spoke to Judy a few weeks after that session. In the intervening time, she had had new x-rays that came back with the following reading: No calculi. The stone was completely gone!

ACID REFLUX

"For a long time I experienced the constant threat and misery of acid reflux disease."

Roy, a vital and distinguished gentleman, came to me at age 89. He had suffered with acid reflux for a long time, including a dreadful burning in his throat and stomach, and an appalling taste in his mouth. He had to be very careful about what and when he ate and would often be awakened during the night with great pain and discomfort. Roy's medical doctor had prescribed endless amounts of Gaviston pills for the symptoms but offered no actual remedy. The pills did little to relieve the unrelenting pain, discomfort, and burning sensation. The acidic, acrid taste in his mouth continued to be intolerable.

I asked Roy if he would like to have a healing session right there and then, where he stood chatting outside. He readily agreed (although he was concerned about what the neighbors might say!) I stood next to him and put my hand on his solar plexus and on his back. Right away, the energies began and I started to feel the familiar heat. We stood there for about 10 minutes and then we were complete.

The next day Roy reported that he had slept right through the entire night and that the burning feeling and taste was totally gone. In just one 10-minute session the condition completely disappeared!

It has been over a year now and Roy continues to be free of all the former acid reflux pain and discomfort and can pretty well eat whatever he likes.

"I'm overjoyed now to report that after just a few minutes with Philip, my discomfort has all but vanished!! It has truly been a life-changing experience for me. Philip is a miracle worker!"

SHOULDER AND NECK PAIN

"I don't know what you did, but my pain has been completely cured."

Whitney attended a special restorative yoga class of about a dozen people, where I was able to spend about six or seven minutes with each participant in a healing class setting. She reported that, in just those few minutes, I was able to completely heal her long-standing shoulder and neck problems.

KNEE PROBLEMS

"I can hardly walk, I can't skate. All my practice will be wasted."

Mary was a pre-teen figure skater. She had been unable to skate for some time due to a nasty fall. Her parents took her to physical therapists and specialists throughout the Toronto area with no success. Now, her father brought her to me, literally carrying her in. I spoke with Mary as she lay on a couch while her dad sat outside by the window enjoying the afternoon sun. As I spoke to her and put my hands on her knees and legs, she drifted off into a deep relaxation. After about an hour she was complete and said she felt as if she had been on a wonderful vacation and gave a vivid account of all kinds of beautiful colors while in this dream-like state. The next day, her parents were dumbfounded as they watched her perform skating jumps with ease.

Mary said, "After I saw you, I could walk again, and the very next day I was actually doing figure skating jumps for the first time in five months. I am not going to miss the nationals after all. Thank you so much!"

TEETH AND ROOT CANAL

"I have terrible tooth pain. Another root canal will cost me thousands!"

Over the years, Clare had had a number of painful and expensive root canals. Recently, the pain began again and her dentist recommended yet another. Clare had received a number of healing sessions from me for other health and wellness concerns and, when I asked her, said she was open to trying some healing on her jaw and teeth as well.

As she lay back deeply relaxed on her couch, I gently cradled her right jaw and touched her lower molars. After about an hour, we were complete and the next day, the pain had gone. Clare cancelled the root canal procedure with her dentist and is problem-free to this day. In just one session we eliminated the pain and we eliminated the issue.

FOOT PROBLEMS

"I'm afraid my life is over."

Hanna had severe foot problems and was not able to walk properly. Her job of 25 years required her to be mobile and on her feet all day so this issue was completely debilitating. When we met, I spoke to Hanna and explained to her about the strength and power of non-physical energies. I touched her arm and heart. After that the pain in Hanna's feet went away.

Hanna says, "I thought my life was over because I could not walk. If I couldn't walk I would not be able to work. Now I can walk pain-free again. You are my savior! I am so grateful. Thank you!"

CHEST PAIN AND FIBROID TUMORS

"All my life I have been in pain. Now, I feel wonderful."

Kaitlin is a nurse. She had experienced severe and unrelenting pain in her upper chest all her life. There was no known medical cause found, even after every type of medical test had been conducted. She also had dreadful pain in her lower abdomen due to two inoperable fibroid tumors. After her first healing session, the pain in her upper chest left completely. After the second, the intolerable pain in her lower abdomen disappeared.

Kaitlin says, "Now I feel wonderful! Thank you!"

There are, of course, many, many more anecdotes covering almost every imaginable type of malady, but this is all the room we have for now. As the authority on energy healing, I hope that you have found this chapter to be helpful as an introduction to such an expansive metaphysical topic. The concepts may be new to you, although the principles have always been used, in every part of the world, throughout history.

If you feel that I may be able to assist you or a loved one, please call me in Toronto at 416-447-9550. If there is a good fit with us and we do work together, I will visit you in the privacy of your own home and I will commit to working with you until you are completely well again. In the meantime, may blessings of Love and Light always be upon you.

Thank you for your interest! You can learn more at www.PhilipYoungHealer.com

The Modern Healer

HERMAN SIU & MARTIN SIU

Good health is a God-given right; it's our birthright. Yet, while we have made huge technological advances to facilitate cross-planet communication in real-time, we haven't been as progressive in keeping ourselves healthy.

We may be living longer but, tragically, children are dying from cancers, diabetes is on the rise, and young adults are suddenly getting heart attacks. Chronic fatigue, depression, and anxiety assail us. We rely on drugs to fix our health problems and we spend billions of dollars on prescriptions that may alleviate the symptoms but leave the root cause untouched. In our fast-paced societies, we have lost the connection with nature and the natural elements that make up our bodies. Surely, there is an alternative way to heal ourselves, or even to prevent disease from occurring in the first place.

The long and short of it is that we don't have to drop out of society and reside in the woods to live happier and healthier lives. The answer to good health and longevity lies right at our fingertips – in the air we breathe, the foods we eat, and water we drink. That's the best prescription for the Modern Healer, and these are the guiding principles we use in our healing practice. As 5th and 6th generation healers immersed in traditions that date back to ancient Chinese Shaolin practices, we adhere to the disciplined and holistic approach of our forefathers.

We believe that a body in full balance has everything it needs to fight off disease, stay and look young, and be active and involved, regardless of the biological age. This belief has been supported by patient outcomes through successive centuries of practice by the healers in our family. We share this knowledge with you to empower you as a Modern Healer, so that you may take control of and assume responsibility for your own health and be the expert in your own healing and wellness journey.

To be empowered as a Modern Healer, you must first understand the core concepts of energy or Qi (chi) as defined by ancient Chinese healing texts.

Dr. Paul Unschuld, a highly-regarded authority on Chinese medicine and multi-book author said, "The core Chinese concept of qi bears no resemblance to the Western concept of 'energy'. We perceive that there is a knowledge gap in the current understanding of eastern medicine in the western world. Mindful of the wisdom suggested by the Chinese proverb, "A journey of a thousand miles begins with a single step," we have written this chapter as our first step towards bridging that divide.

There are three primary components to balance Qi. Qi is a fundamental power underlying all of nature, and it is a vital life force that runs through our body. There are three primary components to balance our Qi. The first component to boosting our Qi is the air we breathe, the second is the food we eat, and the third is the water we drink.

AIR GIVES LIFE

Almost all of life needs oxygen to survive. We take in oxygen from our surroundings to harness energy and use it to power the inner workings of our bodies.

In the Huangdi Neijing, the ancient Chinese foundation medical text, the lungs breathe in what's known as, da qi, or "great qi.". Once we breathe in the air, the lungs extract the Qi from the da qi. Based on this understanding, we perceive that Qi relates to life-sustaining oxygen.

What is the secret to having great Qi? It is the harmonization of the mind, body, and spirit.

In martial arts, we use our mind to harness Qi by controlling our breath. We use our body to breathe, and we put our bodies through constant practice to master our Qi. Once it has been mastered, the Qi can be at our fingertips in a moment's notice. We call it in this form the spirit.

Viewed from this perspective, it's simple to make the most of living and get the best use of your life. The first step to taking back control of your health is by learning to breathe correctly.

Notice, right this moment, how you are breathing. Are you breathing from your diaphragm or the stomach, or are you taking in quick snatches of air? The majority of us take shallow breaths because we have forgotten how to breathe deeply and fully, and the only time we do so is when we are in yoga or meditation. Having become a society of superficial breathers, we are not benefitting from the fact that 70% of the toxins in our bodies are released through breath. By breathing shallowly, we are shortchanging ourselves because hypoxia, or insufficient oxygen in the body's cells, has been linked to degenerative diseases.

Remember, breath equals life and a long breath enhances a long life. Breathing correctly is your first responsibility as a Modern Healer.

FOOD FOR HEALING

The second primary component to balance our Qi is food.

The ancient Greek physician, Hippocrates, who is widely known as the "Father of Medicine", is quoted as saying "Let food be thy medicine and medicine be thy food." Fast forward several centuries; Dr. Roger J. Williams, who discovered the B-vitamin, said in 1971, "The human body heals itself and nutrition provides the resources to accomplish the task." The Chinese are well known to eat their food in its season. For example, no watermelon is eaten in winter since it grows in the hot summer climate.

It is empowering to discover that we need look no further than our own gardens and our kitchens to find healing nutrition that supports health for our family. By making healthy food choices, we ensure that we age gracefully and live out the rest of the twilight years harmoniously and peacefully, without the blight of Alzheimer's, dementia, or other failing diseases.

> *"So many people spend their health gaining wealth & then have to spend their wealth to regain their health."* - Chinese proverb

Our philosophy is that, with right air, right food and right water (in this order), you detoxify naturally, without having to go on rigid short-term fasts.

With the right balance of foods that are appropriate to your body type, you'll get rid of excess fat and flab, find the correct body weight, be brimming over with energy, have the mental clarity to solve challenges with ease, and be in love with your life.

If you're tired of feeling frustrated, angry, depressed, unsure, overweight, tired, and in despair, look to your shopping list, refrigerator and kitchen closets for the culprits. Are they full of processed foods and refined sugars? Are you eating natural grains, green leafy vegetables and fresh fruit?

In this chapter, we'll draw on healing secrets that we share with our clients in our Toronto-based clinic. We'll discuss the major foods that prevent inflammation, help you recover from cuts and wounds, and help detoxify the system.

But for the Modern Healer, the first line of defense is maintaining a healthy pH balance. Acid is corrosive and is the biggest culprit of many degenerative and deadly diseases. It's true that some acid is needed in the body. The stomach uses it to break down the food we eat into macronutrients such as proteins, fats and carbohydrates, and micronutrients such as vitamins and minerals that it may be easily absorbed by the body. But most typical diets are packed with sugar, animal proteins, and processed foods.

WHY PH BALANCE IS CRUCIAL TO GOOD HEALTH

The pH is a measure of acidity or alkalinity. The billions of cells that make up our bodies need an alkaline environment to function, to stay healthy, and to regenerate. Too much acid in our bodies creates ripe conditions for the growth of bacteria, yeast, fungus, viruses, mold and other diseases. Cells that are starved of oxygen are unable to regenerate. Once starved, they are unable to repair damage or rid the body of noxious chemicals and toxins. In time, the cells die; research now points out that cancer is the result of an over-acidic body. An ideal balance for our bodies is measured between a pH of 7.2 – 7.4. You can measure this by dipping pH testing strips into a sample of saliva or urine. An acidic body will produce a pH reading of less than 7.2, which means there is a lack of oxygenation at the cellular level. Your body may even create more fat cells to store the corrosive acid, leading to unwanted weight gain. If the body is malnourished or lacking any Alkaline minerals, it goes in search of calcium to optimize the pH level, and extracts calcium from your bones (joints), teeth and tissues which in turn leaves the bones weak. Calcium is one of the most important alkaline minerals as it increases the oxygen level in the blood. This calcium depletion results in arthritis and osteoporosis. In the initial stages of over-acidity, you may suffer from joint pains, headaches, and weight gain. In an acidic state, the body is trying to expel excess acid through your skin, causing muscle cramps, eczema, acne, swelling, irritation, and general aches and pains. People in this state get grouchier and irritable, and they age faster than those with a balanced pH body. Other so-called modern diseases linked to an acidic body include diabetes, osteoarthritis, acid reflux, irritable bowel syndrome, premature aging, muscle and chronic fatigue, bone loss and osteoporosis.

> *"The only way to keep good health is to eat what you don't want, drink what you don't like, & do what you'd rather not"* -Chinese proverb

GETTING YOUR PH BALANCE RIGHT THROUGH FOODS

Our experience has shown that a balanced diet should be 85-90% alkaline and 10-15% acidic. Body functions and hand-eye coordination work at their optimal state at these levels. It's better for the body to be slightly alkaline than it is to be slightly acidic. Now that we understand why the pH balance is the first line of defense and why it's crucial to maintain the correct pH balance, let's explore quickly what foods contribute to a more alkaline state and more acidic state. A food is classified as alkaline or acidic according to its mineral content. Alkaline-forming foods contain more minerals such as calcium, magnesium, manganese, iron, and potassium. Some acid-promoting minerals include phosphorous, copper, and sulfur. Carbonated drinks are acid forming because they are loaded with sugar and phosphorus, which can lead to weight gain. Have a healthy serving of kale or broccoli instead, which nourishes your body with helpful calcium and magnesium for bone and muscle health. Alkaline foods include apples, apricots, cantaloupes, cauliflower, broccoli, kale, almonds, chestnuts and walnuts. The complete list is much longer and we will examine the healing qualities of alkaline-based nutrition in the section under Anti-Inflammation Foods. Acidic foods include ice-cream, manufactured processed foods with refined sugar, meat, fish, poultry, and eggs. This is not to say that all fruits and vegetables are alkaline. Some are in fact very acidic. Acidic vegetables include corn, onions, and garlic. In the fruit category will fall cranberries, blueberries, and currants. As you grow older, it's harder to expel the acid that is in your body. The longer acid exists, the more it will congeal and the more it will attack your cells and immune system. Acidic conditions manifest one illness at a time. Symptoms include arthritis, muscle fatigue, and body aches. At the point that you are weakest is when you're most prone to infections and diseases because infections live off acidic waste products. At our clinic, we will examine the root cause of your health problems, not just the symptoms. We will customize a holistic healing plan drawing on our experience and expertise to restore you to the right balance, homeostasis, so you may live your life in joy and harmony.

"Tell me and I'll forget; show me and I may remember; involve me and I'll understand" - Chinese proverb

ALKALINE AND ANTI-INFLAMMATION FOODS

Inflammation is a natural body response to injury. You bruise when you hit your shin against a table leg or when you sprain an ankle. Chronic inflammation, if undetected, can result in debilitating illnesses such as heart disease, cancer, diabetes, arthritis, and Alzheimer's. Fried and processed foods, as well as foods that contain trans-fat, increase the risk of inflammation. We've mentioned that alkaline foods prevent inflammation, and these are ordinary fruits, vegetables, and herbs that you can find in your refrigerator, spice cabinet, and even in your own garden. There are many creative ways to prepare these foods for a delicious, nutritious, beneficial anti-inflammation diet/alkaline diet. Here is a small list of foods to keep your body in balance and in good health.

Avocados: they contain healthy fats, phyto-proteins, vitamins, minerals and dietary fiber that is sorely lacking in the western societies. Low in sugar content, avocados may help to lower cholesterol levels, and increase resistance to diabetes, coronary heart disease, stroke and cancer, while promoting a healthy body weight and body mass index (BMI). Avocados are best eaten fresh.

Bamboo shoots: which is not a common vegetable on the western table, were identified by the Compendium of Materia Medica, the most comprehensive medical book in the history of traditional Chinese Medicine. Bamboo shoots promote the circulatory system, supplementing the body's natural energy, and are recommended as a daily dish. A traditional forest vegetable in Chinese diets for 2,500 years, nutrient-rich bamboo shoots are being shown in modern research to help prevent cancer, and to aid in weight loss, digestion, and the appetite.

Bamboo shoots are rich in essential amino acids and fatty acids and, because of their low sugar content, they are useful for treating hypertension, hyperlipemia, and hyperglycemia.

Broccoli: just about all vegetables are good, but some are more alkaline than others. Broccoli counts among the latter as it is rich in important vitamins such as A, C, K, B-complex and minerals including iron, zinc, and phosphorus. Broccoli is also rich in phytonutrients, which are natural chemicals that help protect plants and prevent disease in our bodies.

Broccoli helps to prevent osteoarthritis, reduces the risk of cancer, and has been shown to help reverse diabetes and heart damage. Broccoli is best lightly steamed or gently stir-fried; overcooking will neutralize its benefits.

Cabbage: A source of Vitamins K, C, B6, folate, and thiamine. Cabbage is also a source of iodine to support the health of the brain and the nervous system. This vegetable, which is a staple in Chinese kitchens around the world, helps to lower cholesterol and is rich in glucosinolates that are shown to have cancer prevention properties.

Carrot: Raw or cooked, carrots are a rich source of Vitamins A and C, calcium and iron, and the anti-oxidant beta-carotene that gives the vegetable its orange colour. In addition, carrots contain fibre, Vitamins K and E, potassium, folate, manganese, magnesium, zinc, and some phosphorus. Carrots improve our vision, delay aging, help with regulating blood sugar, improve digestion, and help prevent cancer. There is a side note to add: overconsumption of carrots can be toxic so, if you start turning orange, you may want to cut back on your carrot intake!

Cauliflower: The cauliflower is packed with vitamins such as B1, B2, B3,

B5, B6, B9, C and K, as well as being rich in omega 3, fatty acids, fibre, manganese, and potassium. Apart from delivering powerful antioxidants, cauliflower is a healthy source of protein and fibre, it enhances the body's ability to detoxify, reduces the risk of inflammation and the incidence of cancer. Cauliflower is best lightly cooked through a simple sauté.

Spinach: Spinach is widely acknowledged to be rich in vitamins and minerals such as magnesium, iron, copper, calcium, potassium, and zinc. The dark green spinach is packed with anti-oxidants and health-promoting phyto-nutrients. If you're low in iron, spinach helps to make up the deficit. It is an aid in the management of diabetes, and works towards lowering high blood pressure and improving bone health. Spinach is best eaten lightly steamed, quickly boiled or sautéed.

Ginger: Mankind's historic cure-all, ginger is rich in anti-oxidants, vitamins and minerals, and also contains omega-3 and omega-6. Shown to be anti-inflammatory, anti-cancer, anti-nausea, and a powerful anti-oxidant, it greatly boosts the immune system. A versatile root, ginger can be chewed fresh, steamed, boiled in water to make tea, or grated and added to sautéed dishes.

The state in which it is consumed will affect its benefits greatly. Fresh ginger root fights the common cold, coughs, and asthma, while dried ginger root is better against abdominal pain, cold limbs, and rheumatism. If you were to use the fresh root for rheumatism, the condition will worsen but, fresh or dried, it is effective in preventing or stopping vomiting and diarrhea. Large quantities of fresh ginger are not recommended for those with high blood pressure, inflammatory bowel disease, ulcers, or intestinal blockage, and should be used sparingly if you suffer from gallstones. Excessive consumption can cause a person to break out in a rash as an allergic reaction and may also lead to heartburn, bloating, gas, belching, and even some nausea. From ginger root, we'll move on to alkaline-forming fruit and herbs to round up our short list of recommended foods. Remember, some foods are mildly acidic and some are weak acidic foods. Not all acidic foods are tarred with the same brush, but the worst offenders include processed foods, sugar, tomatoes, onions, garlic, dairy, and vinegar.

Apricot: the fruit and the seeds are effective alkaline-forming foods. Packed with iron and protein, apricots are good for quenching thirst and fighting asthma. The seeds from the bitter apricot heal coughs, sore throats, and constipation, as does the sweet apricot seed. But those suffering from asthma should eat only the bitter apricot seed, or the condition will worsen. Laetrile, a naturally occurring substance found in the kernels, has been increasingly promoted to help in cancer treatment. The apricot kernels have been documented to help fight against tumors as far back as 502 AD. The apricot oil has been used as far back as 17th century England to fight swellings, tumors, and ulcers

Peppermint: a herb with healing benefits dating back to ten thousand years in the past, peppermint is commonly used to fight inflammation. It soothes abdominal pain, indigestion, irritable bowels and bloating, and prevents nausea and vomiting. It is a popular healing food for the common colds that are accompanied by headaches, sore throat and thick phlegm. However, if you are suffering a common cold but have a runny nose, cold limbs and diarrhea, peppermint is not that effective. Although it is commonly thought of as an herb or a spice, it is actually cool and pungent, and should not be used daily. Those suffering from anemia or low blood pressure should use only as directed.

"Health is the greatest gift, Contentment is the greatest treasure, Confidence is the greatest friend, Enlightenment is the greatest bliss." -Chinese proverb

FOODS TO ACCELERATE HEALING OF CUTS AND WOUNDS

Skin is the biggest organ in our bodies, and we tend to take it for granted because small nicks heal quickly. However, there are times when there is a deep cut or wound from an accident or from surgery when extra support is required for the connective tissue to regenerate. Connective tissue is different from most other tissues because it is made not so much of cells, but from protein, notably collagen, fibres encased in a unique covering called a fascia. To boost your ability to heal quickly from cuts and wounds, look for foods with these four pivotal nutrients and minerals.

Vitamin C: Vitamin C assists in forming collagen to repair the connective tissue in the blood vessels, cartilage, muscles, and in the bones. Good sources of Vitamin C include fruits such as guava, kiwi, strawberries, and papaya. Vegetables include red and green sweet peppers, Brussels sprouts, broccoli, cauliflower, and sweet potatoes.

Vitamin A: Some of the foods mentioned in the category above will be useful for sourcing Vitamin A because they are rich beta-carotene that is converted into fully active Vitamin A. This vitamin serves many functions. It promotes growth, maintains the immune system, and supports vision. Other Vitamin A rich foods are sweet potatoes, pumpkins, carrots, spinach, turnip greens, and cantaloupe.

Flavonoids: These are a group of pigments that give plants their colour but are compounds that have been discovered to have anti-oxidant properties that are more powerful against a wider range of oxidants than the traditional antioxidants. They help the body detoxify, reduce inflammation, and prevent and reduce damage at the cellular level. Within this grouping, it's the flavonoid called catechin, which is found in great abundance in tea leaves, that is thought to inhibit the growth of cancerous cells. In addition to green, black, and oolong teas, flavonoids are also found in dark coloured berries, bananas, all citrus fruits, parsley, gingko biloba, and cocoa with chocolate content exceeding 70%.

Zinc: This mineral repairs damaged tissues and aids in healing wounds by generating proteins and other genetic material, boosts cell division andcollagen formation, and regenerates tissue, all of which are crucial to wound repair. It boosts the system, develops and activates the T-cells that fight off infection. Zinc is found in vegetables, nuts and seeds such as asparagus, bamboo shoots, Brussels sprouts, okra, potatoes, pumpkin, Swiss chard, lima beans, peas, pine nuts, cashews, pumpkin, and sunflower seeds.

KEEPING YOUR BRAIN HEALTHY

Fernando Gómez-Pinilla, professor of neurosurgery and physiological science in UCLA, describes food as a "pharmaceutical compound that affects the brain".

Studies conducted by him show that the brain is highly susceptible to oxidation damage, so foods that are high in antioxidants protect the brain cells from damage and dysfunction.

Omega-3 fatty acids: These fatty acids support the plasticity of the synapses in the brain that affect critical functions. These include learning and memory, fighting off depression, bipolar disorders, schizophrenia, and attention-deficit disorders. The particularly important omega-3 fatty acid is docosahexaenoic acid or DHA, which reduces oxidative damage, improves synapse plasticity, and is needed in the brain's cell membranes. Omega-3s are found abundantly in walnuts, avocados, flaxseed, chia, and kiwi fruit. Though typically recommended as a desirable source of fatty acids, we take a strong stand against salmon as a source of omega-3s. The oceans are filled with toxins such as mercury, dioxin, and more recently radiation, and seafood is filled with these dangerous elements. In our annals of healing, this leads to mental and neurological disorders such as dementia, Alzheimer's, and multiple sclerosis. It is much safer and healthier to find the fatty acids in nuts and fruit.

Folic Acid: The brain needs sufficient folic acid for its functions, and folate deficiency leads to depression and cognitive impairment. Combining folic acid with other B vitamins has been effective in slowing the rate of age-related decline in cognitive function, and in preventing dementia. Folic acid is found in green leafy vegetables such as spinach, asparagus, romaine, dried or fresh beans and peas, as well as in avocados, beets, broccoli, peanuts, sunflower seeds, honeydew melons, cantaloupes, bananas, raspberries, and grapefruits.

FOODS FOR DETOXIFICATION

In our view, a good detoxification is much more than a spring-cleaning. It's like a good oil change – you take out the gunk and replace it with good, clean nutrients that power the body.

We design tailored and customized detoxification programs that both cleanse and support your system. The concept behind our programs is that it's not enough just to flush out the toxins with a juice cleanse. Instead, you need to simultaneously put back nourishment and support that will revitalize and energize the organs and the immune system.

With that being said, the key organ that is most prone to work overload is the liver. The liver supports almost every organ in the body. It is the second largest organ in the body, and any alcohol or drugs taxes it severely. When that happens, the liver performs less than optimally, leading to an accumulation of toxins that in turn cause chronic illnesses. Natural detoxification foods and herbs are best prescribed after a complete diagnosis to know what is best for your body constitution.

Natural diuretics: Foods that flush the body of toxins are essential to a good detoxification or to counteract the effects of an unhealthy lifestyle. Among natural diuretics are watercress, dandelions in the form of tea, celery, and cabbage, in which is found the antioxidant glutathione to improve the liver's detoxifying function. Be advised that natural diuretics must be used with care; the amount and type to be consumed will depend on your individual body type and constitution.

THE TRUTH ABOUT WATER

The third component to balance our Qi is water.

Water covers 71% of the Earth's surface and is vital to all forms of life. Your body ranges between 50-75% of water as body composition varies according to gender and fitness level, because adipose tissue contains less water than lean tissue. Suffering from fuzzy short-term recall, having problems with mental math or reading small print? Those are signs of dehydration. Be careful in your choice of what you drink. Tap water, sodas, and coffee are all acidic. Our rule is 8x8. We recommend drinking at least eight 8-oz. glasses of water a day to neutralize the acid in the bloodstream for better metabolism and more efficient absorption of nutrients. For those looking for alkaline water, we prefer AquaHydrate, which has a pH of 9+, but only use as directed.

"When you are sick of sickness, you are no longer sick." -Chinese proverb

BE AN EMPOWERED MODERN HEALER

We hope this journey into the healing properties of good nutrition will empower you to make the right choices. Whether it is to give you more energy, get you thinking clearly, accelerate recovery from illnesses, or to age with grace, the choice to eat well and live well rests in your hands. You may find the way ahead difficult and you may need a boost to get you started on the right footing. You may have inexplicable aches, pains, or chronic colds and allergies that just simply refuse to go away. Just changing your diet is not enough to get you on the healing path. Whether you seek preventative care or deep healing, we have the alternative modalities to help you with the healing transformation.

The body is a finely-tuned mechanism. It works until it is out of balance and, even then, it seeks to right itself until the imbalance has buried itself too deeply. Once it does, we are assailed with all forms of diseases and ailments, some too deep to be cured with just nutrition.

As practitioners, we tap into the secrets of our forefathers, into healing practices that have been refined and polished and provided to thousands and thousands of patients through six generations of healers. These are intricate and sophisticated methods of diagnosis, healing, and remedies that are the result of centuries of observation and practice that have withstood the tests of time and the tests of western medicine.

We are deeply immersed in a culture of healing and we drill down to the causes of disease and illness by identifying patterns of disharmony in your body. Our methods are gentle and non-invasive, and we examine not just the visible symptoms, but also take into account the subtle, intangible forces that make up all life. As healers deeply ingrained in a compassionate practice, we examine the physical, mental, emotional, and spiritual aspects because the body, mind, and spirit are inseparable. When you consult with us, you benefit not just from our knowledge and experience, but also from the cumulative wisdom and healing of our medical ancestors.

Martin and Herman are 5th and 6th generation healers steeped in Chinese healing traditions preserved through a lineage that dates back to Shaolin Buddhist principles. As father and son, they run their Toronto-based clinic on a mission to bridge the ancient and modern worlds to take healing to the next level. They seek to bring the body's energies to balance through a holistic and compassionate approach to healing. They customize nutritional plans and draw on modalities such as acupuncture and Tong Ren, a specialized energy therapy, Qi Gong breathing and exercise routines to empower the patient in the healing journey. They are currently co-authoring an upcoming book in response to overwhelming demand from their clients. It will be a thorough look at the beneficial properties, compounds, antioxidants, and micronutrients found in food, and will include ancient breathing and exercise secrets that assist in the healing process. Get more information at http://omaniclinic.com.

How To Gain Abundant Wealth

KAY EVE

This advice is aimed at two groups of people – first, those who heard the name of God but have not taken further action and second, those from a practising Christian background who have lapsed.

If, however, you are an atheist then the teachings described here cannot help you. I wish it were otherwise, but I cannot change how the universe is. Without belief, you cannot have God's spiritual help in your search for wealth and wellbeing. Without belief, you must rely on only human knowledge to see you through the difficult times.

The issue is that Christian teachings are haunted by two very wrong ideas. Firstly, the notion that suffering is good for you and that we must each "bear our own cross". One such example is that Mother Theresa of Calcutta refused medicine to patients in her "hospitals" because of the belief that suffering was "good for the soul." This was not the Middle Ages, but only 20 years ago, showing how deeply embedded the idea that "suffering is good, yet pleasure is dangerous" still is within Christianity even to this day. I won't deal with this idea here extensively other than to say that there are many churches that will tell you the good news, that God wants us to be happy – and what's wrong with being happy? I advise you to visit an evangelical church. The worst that can happen is you'll have a good laugh.

The second wrong impression within Christianity is that it is wrong to long for material gains. Jesus famously overturned money changers' tables in the Temple. He said "it is easier for a camel to go through the eye of a needle than for someone who is rich to enter the kingdom of God". I hope to show that what God hates isn't making money, but acquiring it dishonestly or hoarding it all to yourself. Instead, Christian teaching encourages us to live a comfortable life with your loved ones and to do good with the excess. This interpretation is often ridiculed as "praying for money", particularly by spiritual people who I want to reach. Good people also deserve to succeed! So I ask you to keep an open mind, and to give me benefit of a doubt and give careful consideration to what I have to say.

I'm certainly not saying that the Bible tells you that if you ask for gifts from God then they will just fall into your lap! Many of the good things that Gods gives us are quite unasked for – sometimes things will just come miraculously. However, what the teachings say is that if you ask, He will help you to help yourself. You will have to supply the hard work for financial success or personal happiness, but God will be right by your side.

Read on and discover God's love for us all. I know in my heart that if we start looking closely, we can find messages of encouragement that God gives mankind, messages that have mostly been covered over or shunned. I'm here to try and bring out the truth, that God wants us to know His desire for everyone to be happy and have a meaningful, fulfilling life.

And so, I thank God every day for everything that was created directly by Him and indirectly by humans in our world. I am so grateful to be here amongst all of you today.

THE GREAT DISCOVERY

When we think of our galaxy, we know that it is shaped just like a fried egg with the yellow yolk in the middle and a disc of white surrounding it. In the outer edge of the disc is our sun, with one of its planets that we call Earth, which is found to be a safe place for all living things.

During the 19th and 20th centuries, scientists gradually discovered how the universe and the earth formed and evolved. The human race had already been running around planet earth for thousands of years, living and breeding on the planet quite successfully when at peace but killing each other in times of war. Those ancient people had no knowledge of how the earth was formed, but still some of them knew the wealth teachings, and so they came to be wealthy and successful.

If you look at the world's religions today, the only faiths that teach us how to live with Abundant Wealth are the teaching of the Torah for Jews and the Old and New Testaments for Christians. The Abundant Wealth teachings were recorded in all the books we call the Bible, within which one can acquire the keys to unlock wealth and happiness.

More and more people are now searching for words of guidance from the sages of old and from modern businessmen and businesswomen alike. One may not realise that the roots of the valuable teaching from modern day "coaches" actually originate from Christian doctrine. Most people in our modern world do not know how to use and apply the keys successfully to their own lives. But through keeping in mind these teachings and keys, it is possible to achieve your goals and attain wealth, success, happiness and wellbeing.

The only thing that can maintain an abundance of wealth, success and prosperity is God. He has played the biggest part in all our lives whether we realise it or not. People can say they don't believe in God, but if they do, they won't have access to His teachings for success. A lot of people believe in other religions, but abundance only comes down to us from the most powerful, the most almighty, the most gracious and the most merciful one called God. The truth is that there is only one key in the universe and God himself has the key. By praising and asking God for His Abundant Wealth's codes you will learn how to apply the codes for yourself and become successful in every aspect of your life.

The simple question is how to become wealthy? If you believe in God, you will discover these Abundant Wealth's codes and be able to use these codes to unlock for yourself whatever your heart desires, in your personal life, business, work or family. When you have learned this, you will have learned the secret of one of the most satisfying experiences of life. You may say "Well, that's okay for those who already know God, but what about people that do not know or have never heard of God before?"

If you happen to be later, that is ok; it is very easy to join this group of enlightened. By way of illustration, I will call it a club. As you already know, if you aren't a member of a certain club, you cannot receive the access, knowledge or privileges which members can. To be in God's presence is like being in God's club just like the other Christian or religious sects' clubs.

With God we have free will to choose to worship Him or not. That is your personal choice. God does not need anything from you except to receive your sincere love and your worship. God does not want you to sacrifice anything to

Him. He has already sacrificed his own beloved son Jesus Christ for us over two thousand years ago.

Firstly, you need to believe that there is such a thing as the Supreme Being who is commonly referred to as "God", with His own special holy names by which He would prefer to be called. Without this belief, you will not have your wealth key's codes to work. If you do not believe that God exists, then why in the universe or on earth would you expect any of His Abundant Wealth's codes to work for you?

Secondly, endeavour to believe that God has the power to grant you your Wealth codes to unlock the doors of the universe and give you all aspects of success and abundant wealth. God can indeed be reached directly, for there is no distance between Him and His Son.

If you are not in God's club you are an outsider, you will not receive full wisdom to understand all of God's instructions laid out before your eyes. As Jesus has told his disciples in Mark's Gospel,

Mark 4:12 Jesus said, *"When they see what I do, they will learn nothing. When they hear what I say, they will not understand. Otherwise, they will turn to me and be forgiven."*

The "forgiven" word here means to be freed from wrong decisions, wrong choices, etc. So your faith in Jesus will make these mysterious passages, the codes, clear.

EVERYTHING IS POSSIBLE

First you need to do everything physically and mentally possible to make a good connection with God!

When we discover that we are known and understood by God, it can be a very profound and moving experience. Sometimes your spouse or best friend may know or understand you on the surface, but deep down you may feel like you are alone. And yet no matter how well you are known or understood by others, no one can understand you better than God himself. As King David has put it;

Psalm 139:1-4 NIV
"O Lord, you have searched me and you know me. You know when I sit and when I rise; you perceive my thoughts from afar. You discern my going out and my lying down; you are familiar with all my ways. Before a word is on my tongue; you know it completely. O Lord."

If you believe that God exists in the world like the ancient people of past times did, then you will want to worship the Almighty for the successes in your life. But how can you actually get a real and intimate connection to Him? The sincerity of your heart is the key to success.

Three steps to Calmness:

1. Find solitude with God, away from other people and distractions. By shutting out the sights and sounds around, you will make it easy to tune in with God.

2. Find a comfortable position, select a chair or a corner of your bed. Go to the same place at the same time in the same position every day. Consistency is of the utmost importance.

3. Before you begin, relax and take a few deep breaths. Let your mind be quiet and your body relaxed. When your mind quietens, you may know the conscious presence of God that says "Be still and know that I am God." Psalm 46:10

Now you are ready to start making a connection.

Three Steps to Listening:

1. The first step of prayer is to praise God, such as by citing the Lord's Prayer as in Matthew 6: 9-13. Let your prayer begin by praising God and you will soon find yourself in a frame of mind with Him.

2. Let some positive thinking and praying enter your mind. The secret of success is thinking and believing positively, and the same is true in prayer.

3. Ask Him to speak to you and tell Him about the things that matter to you. Whatever problems or difficulties you have, you can rely on Him for comfort, stability and the material things that the world has to offer. Once you have things off your chest, remain quite still and relaxed and listen!

By modern standards in the developed world, very few of us are really suffering. The atheists down the street will probably have all they need and live physically as well as you, perhaps even a little better. Yet, if you ask God, you will receive more blessings than they ever will and be in a better place with a better quality of life, with all the things you ask for that can be truly beneficial to you.

EXPECTING THE UNEXPECTED

Secondly you must believe that he has the power to help us and wants to help us all!

When you have asked God for the things I have described above, one final step remains - the "receiving in advance", or the assurance that your prayer will be answered. You need to thank Him and to strongly assert your confidence that He is going to provide the answer to your request. Filling your heart with positive thoughts will help to ensure that God will allow these things to happen.

Yet, how can you be assured that a constant relationship with God will produce answered prayer? The answer lies within the Abundant Wealth codes, within the heart of answered prayer, and within the following everyday Bible verses, such as;

Matthew 17:20
If you have faith as a grain of mustard seed, you shall say unto this mountain, "Remove from here" and it will move. Nothing will be impossible for you." (The "mountain" in this parable of Jesus means one of our life's great crises.)

Matthew 21:22
If you believe, you will receive whatever you ask for in prayer.

Mark 21:24
Therefore, I tell you whatever you ask for in prayer, believe that you have received it and it will be yours.

However, do not mix up the word "Faith" with "Belief". To believe that God can answer and is able to deliver all of the things being asked for in prayer, this is not faith. Everyone can have faith. The prayer of faith means trusting in God to do something but truly believing in God means to know that God is honest and will do what He says He will. It is to believe unhesitatingly that He is on the verge of doing it and that even now, the answer is on the way to you.

Many people also misconceive faith as desire, but this is false. Many people want success, but longing, wanting and desiring success is not faith. Desire, rightly directed, can produce faith and may lead you to faith, but in itself it is not faith. When you have known God intimately, you may experience a genuine re-dedication of your heart, only to be disappointed that your prayer went unanswered. This is because God may judge that the "good" thing was not what you really need at that time. He will give you something else that's good, something that benefits your life.

Faith is a common commodity. Everyone has faith. Atheists have faith that there is no God. Animals and pets have faith in their masters. Children have faith in their parents and we have faith in our Governments to watch over our nation. It is only faith in God through truly believing in Him that will reward you with your heart's desire. As James says in James 1:6-8;.

"But when you ask God, you must believe and not doubt, because he who doubts (unbelief) is like a wave of the sea, blown and tossed by the wind. That man should not think he will receive anything from the Lord, he is a double-minded man, unstable in all he does."

Believing is an act of total trust in God; it doesn't require information, knowledge or certainty – only the free and joyful surrender in His goodness. To help with this, look for the "invisible" gifts of God. They are clearly seen in the many good things that have already happened, things that are usually taken for granted. However, God alone will not change the course of some worldly events. For instance, He doesn't interfere with situations in which people have created chaos around themselves. They must deal with the consequences of their own actions. God is very constant, but for victims caught in the chaos He will turn things around for those who have the absolute trust in Him.

Each code of Abundant Wealth is laid out in the Bible for anyone to read. It has rarely been used before because few pay attention or even try to find out the meaning that God has given freely to everyone. Established religions tell people that praying for money or success is the sin of "avarice", yet churches get rich while their congregations are told to be content with what they have. But who can build a hospital or invent a new medicine without money? It is not the money that is inherently bad; it is the people that do bad things with or for it.

Most modern day sages who have written books about God's wealth codes have hidden the source of these gifts, saying that they come from the universe instead of from God Himself. One can ask for wealth, success, love and happiness until your tongue hangs out, but you will not receive the answer without asking only God himself.

Asking others who pretend to be God for favours will end in disastrous results for you, even if it may appear to be beneficial at first. Many rich and famous people have made deals with others but there is a steep price that must be paid for this false hope. Through Jesus Christ, we have paid already and there is nothing to fear when asking for success, as long as it is done without wickedness or dishonesty.

If you are still skeptical about the wealth key's code then it will not work for you. I wish you good health and happiness, but if you remain doubtful you might as well throw this book away! To have everything that you need and desire you must make a total surrender of your heart, your love and your belief to God, the powerful and the almighty who has created this world and the universe. As is said in Hebrews 11:1-6;

> "Now faith is being sure of what we hope for and certain of what we do not see .... By faith we understand that the universe was formed at God's command, so that what is seen was not made out of what was visible .... And without faith it is impossible to please God, because anyone who comes to him must believe that he exists and that he rewards (Abundant Wealth to) those who earnestly seek him."

THE TRUTH REVEALED

Who is "God" and what's wrong with the idea of a general "Supreme Being"?

God defines Himself as the great lover of mankind, and many Bible verses reveal the depth of this love.

Jeremiah 9:24
"I am the Lord, I show unfailing love, I do justice and right upon the earth; for on this I have set my heart"

Jeremiah 31:3
"I have loved you with an everlasting love; I have drawn you with loving kindness."

Mark 11:29-33
"A new command I give you: Love one another. As I have loved you, so you must love one another."

Most religious texts, Hebrew and Muslim alike, give many names of God in their own Language - seventy-two in Hebrew and up to ninety-nine for Muslims. The only one that God told Moses directly is found in Exodus 33:19. "I will call out my name, Yahweh" ("The Lord"). Even so, there are many other names given to God which reflect the compassion, kindness and generosity He had for different peoples, such as;

Yahweh-Jireh Lord will provide

Yahweh-Rohi Lord is my shepherd

Yahweh-El Shadia	Lord Almighty
Yahweh-Shalom	Lord of peace
Yahweh-Rapha	Lord of healing

Yahweh-El-Olam   Lord everlasting

Yahweh-M'kaddesh   Lord who sanctifies

As mentioned in the Old Testament, no one can see God face-to-face and live to tell, due to his vast and glorious power being too much for our bodies of mere flesh and bone. For this reason, when God appeared to Moses He covered Moses' body with the shadow of His hand.

Exodus 33:19
"I will make all my goodness pass by before you. For I will show mercy to anyone I choose, and I will show compassion to anyone I choose."

Exodus 33:20
"but you may not look directly at my face, for no one may see me and live."

As we know from the Bible, God created the universe, the world and all living things on it. Among these creations was the Sun, which produced the light and heat that God commanded to shine upon the Earth as God had wanted from the beginning.

Genesis 1:1 & 31
"In the beginning God created the heavens and earth...And God said "let there be light."

And so, humans were born on Earth in multitudes, and from them God selected the nation of Israel and the Jewish people to work with Him. Much of the Old Testament tells of God's love towards this nation. Yet men were disobedient and uncaring towards God, turning away to worship frightful and false gods instead. And so the New Testament tells us that God sent his son, Jesus Christ, to be born as a human among us and so that we would love and worship him again. As the Bible says, if we accept that Jesus is our Lord and the son of God, then we become God's adopted children and have the right to call him Father and to ask for his Wealth Keys.

> Matthew 7:11
>
> *Jesus says, "Ask and it will be given to you; seek and you will find; knock and the door will be opened to you.....which of you, if your children ask for bread, will give them a stone.....if you, then, though you are evil, know how to give good gifts to your children, how much more will your Father in heaven give good gifts to those who ask Him."*

So what do we know about God so far? We know we can ask Him for help in all matter of things and that nothing is too big or small for Him to handle. We can ask Him for guidance in all of our problems because He truly cares, and we can also ask him for whatever we desire and it shall be done for us. If we know God intimately and are not happy with our present situation, then we can always ask Him to change it for the better. We must remember that there is no god other than Yahweh-God who proved his love for us by laying down his own son's life for our benefit. The people who get their prayers answered are just simple people like you and I. We must never doubt in Him and we must always rest assured; God is real. He was, He is and He will be in everyone's life.

THE ASKING

But how can you actually go about asking God for Abundant Wealth?

Everything is possible with God for those who love Him. You can trust in God that all that you ask will be fulfilled before you draw your last breath on earth, no matter how long it takes. An example can be seen in Luke Ch. 2 where Simon, the old Jewish prophet who was full of devotion to God, asked that he might meet the Messiah in his own lifetime. God answered his wishes and promised Simon would meet him before he died.

Luke 2:27-29
Led by the spirit, Simon went into the Temple. So when Mary and Joseph came to present the baby Jesus to The Lord as the law required. Simon took the baby Jesus into his arms and praised God, saying "Master, now you are dismissing your servant in peace according to your promise."

It is God's will that his children will possess Abundant Wealth and all that they desire. And so we now need to concentrate on how to build a relationship with God in order to receive his true blessings. Like any relationship, one has to dedicate oneself to make it happen. Though it is common knowledge that true human relationships are not always easy to maintain, it is different with God for he loved you first. He longed for you to love Him back, and it is up to you now to do your part.

There are only a minority of people who have a true belief in God's love and will see a miracle happen to them in their lives. It is hard for most people to love and believe in God, especially being surrounded by modern technology where things must be seen, heard, touched, felt or sensed in order to be real. God and belief in Him have become almost a myth, but the key to finding true belief is to discern God's love in your own life, which can be done in Five Steps.

1. Ask God to step into your heart and reveal his truth to you. You can do this anywhere or any time as long as it feel right to you. Once you have accepted God and Jesus into your heart, you will become an adopted child of God and you can begin building the relationship.

Revelation 3:20
Jesus says; "Look! I stand at the door and knock. If you hear my voice and open the

door, I will come in, and we will share a meal together as friends."

2. Begin worshiping and praising God, whether out loud or silently in your mind. Concentrate on God's love towards your every being. Ask God to clean not only your heart, but your mind, your soul and your entire being. You must create the purest atmosphere to get positive reception of God's intuition and that small voice that speaks directly into your heart.

Nahum 1:7
"The Lord is good, a refuge in times of trouble. He cares for those who trust in him."

3. Study God's word within the Old and New Testaments, asking God for the wisdom to discern the Bible's lessons. The parables are not easily understood the first time they are read, so you must ask for God's help in deciphering them. Only then may you apply them to your personal and professional life, as generations of God's children have done before you.

Mark 4:9-12
"Anyone with ears to hear should listen and understand" … *"You are permitted to understand the secret of the Kingdom of God. But I use parables for everything I say to outsiders, so that the Scriptures might be fulfilled."*

Understand that things which you ask God for can come quickly or slowly depending on how ready you are to receive them. God knows that if he gives them to you when you are not ready, you will lose these gifts or become unable to cope with it. In time, if we use His words and apply them to our lives, we are sure to receive everything that we need or want and we may continue to ask for more.

4. Have faith that God will deliver. You can see how often many people gave up on asking things from God because they could not see any results

coming out of their prayers. Most people have forgotten what the most important part of the prayer is. They forgot to get the most authoritative person to support and speed their request so that it was heard quickly by God. Much like in a court case where you need a proper barrister to work with you to ensure the judge will rule in your favour, it is the same with God. You need your spiritual brother Jesus Christ to help with your prayers so that the Heavenly Father may execute your request. Always ask God for your needs in Jesus' name. But remember, only God knows when the time is right for you to receive his gifts, much like a doctor who knows when to give treatment to his patient. Once you understand all of the above, you can use the Bible Keys and apply them to your personal life.

Isaiah 55:11

God says; "It is the same as my word. I send it out and it always produces fruit. It will accomplish all I want it to, and it will prosper everywhere I send it."

5. Finally, you must give thanks. After you have given your prayer request, you must thank God with all your heart. The more you thank Him, the quicker his blessings will come to you. You must now concentrate on believing one hundred percent in your heart that your request is now heard by God.

There is a final condition that you need to make it work. You must understand that if you have received God's answer to your request, you will now need to get to work on the request you made. You will not receive any kind of blessing that you have not earned, much like the old wives' tale of "help yourself first and God will help you."

Proverbs 10:4

"Lazy hands make a man poor, but diligent hands bring wealth."

Proverbs 22:29
"Be sure you know the condition of your flocks, give careful attention to your herds."

The above five conditions are absolute must-dos if you want your prayer to be answered and to succeed in having God bless you with wellbeing, happiness and success in your life.

Roman 10:11
"As the Scripture says. Anyone who trusts in Him will never be put to shame."

GRATITUDE

Giving thanks is of vital importance, but just Giving to others is also important!

How well do we know the meaning of the word "gratitude"? If you want Abundant Wealth from God, you must be able to change your attitude and behaviour towards what you have been given already.

1 Timothy 6:17
"….. Their trust should be in God, who richly gives us all we need for our enjoyment. Tell them to use their money to do good. They should be rich in good works and generous to those in need. By doing this they will be storing up their treasure as a good foundation for the future so that they may experience true life."

You already know how to trust in God for the things you have asked for. Now you need to know how to act while you are waiting for God to bestow upon you the things you desire. Even if you do not have much, you still need to appreciate what you do have, that which has sustained you until now. You may hate your menial job or be in a boring business, but you must not condemn it. After all, it has kept you afloat until now.

The Key to this is that now you know how to turn things around. While appreciating what sustained you, from its original roots, God will bless it and turn it into a good thing.

Matthew 25:29
Jesus says; "For everyone who has will be given more, and they will have abundance. Whoever does not have, even what they have will be taken from them."

This first sentence above means that your need to be grateful for all the things you currently possess. This appreciation will make them become more important, even if right now they seem worthless to you. The second sentence does not mean that God will take your things away, only that without your appreciate of them, the few resources you have tend to be squandered.

In the physical realm, you may be in a job that you hate but are desperate to leave. You may want God to answer your prayers and to help you out of this predicament. In this instance, while you wait for God to manifest things that you have prayed for, you must learn to imitate God's spiritual realm in order to turn it into your real world.

Romans 8:24
".... But hope that is seen is no hope at all. Who hopes for what he already has? But we hope for what we do not yet have, we wait for it patiently."

If you know the mind of Jesus Christ, you will know that when He was in human form, everything was beautiful and perfect in God's eyes. Jesus was without worry and he was on Earth solely for the purpose of doing God's work. Nothing could harm or touch him because God's power was within him. When he was laid on the cross of crucifixion, it was because Jesus allowed himself to be, in order to fulfill the scriptures and be sacrificed as a lamb of God for all of us.

Therefore, you must have gratitude for Christ's gift because he paid with his life for your sins. You can be free of anxiety, stress, worry, distress and ill health because Jesus removed all those bad things from you. All hardships are of the physical realm; you can be free of these struggles by switching yourself to the spiritual realm.

When you know that God is by your side, your mind will be sharp and focused. No matter what sort of negative thoughts arise, you must not listen to them. They're trying to lure you away from God and all the good things that he has in store for you.

According to Christian teachings, two cosmic broadcast stations – the Light and the Dark – send signals to our brain. Any thought that is loud and clear, which urges you to react to a situation, without a proper plan, that is the enemy – the Dark. But if the thought is barely audible, if it is a soft voice emanating from the recesses of our mind, it is the song of the Light. If you are greeted with a sudden flash of intuition or inspiration, you can be certain it is from the spiritual realm.

The key to taking control of your life is to ignore the loud noise in your head and to take time to concentrate on the small, quiet sounds from God to guide you. When you succeed in blocking out the negative thoughts that manifest themselves as our greedy and selfish egos, the Light signal and all the good thoughts that come along with it are free to fill our minds. The best ideas can come forth at once and without hindrance, and you can see the way to wisdom.

In the Old Testament, during the time that king Ahab ruled in Israel, Ahab did not worship God. He killed all of God's prophets except one, Elijah. Elijah was afraid and asked for God's help. He went into a cave where he spent the night praying and waiting for God's instruction.

1 Kings 11:13

"Go out and stand before me on the mountain" the Lord told him. And as Elijah stood there, the Lord passed by, and a mighty windstorm hit the mountain. It was such a terrible blast that the rocks were torn loose, but the Lord was not in the wind. After the wind there was an earthquake, but the Lord was not in the earthquake. And after the earthquake there was a fire, but the Lord was not in the fire. And after the fire there was the sound of a gentle whisper. ………. And the voice said "What are you (still) doing here, Elijah?"

Thus we can know that the gentle, whispering voice is from God, not the enemy.

You now have all the Abundant Wealth Keys in your hands, and can begin to apply them to all aspects of your life. You can begin to see success in all areas, from your personal and family life, to your professional and business life, and to your community as well.

Finally, remember this. If you care for other human beings like God cares for you, you will continue to receive God's blessing. You will please God if you lend Him a hand, doing charitable work for those less fortunate than you in this world that God has made for us all.

The Secret to Words

JACQUELINE LUCIEN

When you first learned to read, you probably were taught to associate each letter with an object and a sound. It was pretty flat-footed, like "A" is for apple or "B" is for ball. The things your parents or teachers used to illustrate the sound represented by each letter may have made sense to you? Did you ever wonder what the letters originally stood for, *or if they stood for anything* or how someone came up with their specific shapes and curves?

Each letter we use today has a rich and fascinating, multi-layered meaning. Each has a history of associations that make it just about perfect in terms of its shape and design. Just like Chinese and Japanese characters, each letter of the alphabet represents so much more than just a sound — it tells a story and conveys the ancient and original meaning in a powerful way which influences our words today. So, how did these letters that mean so much in our daily lives come to be in the first place?

We all know the old saying that a picture is worth a thousand words. Well, it's true and nowhere more so than when talking about the letters we use to read and write. The alphabet is connected to ancient pictures, and the essence of those pictures comes from both concrete objects and abstract ideas. If a picture is worth a thousand words, and letters (in their ancient essence) are pictures, *what is the worth of one letter? What is the worth of one word?*

THE CREATION OF THE ROMAN ALPHABET

The Roman alphabet (the 26 letters from A to Z used to create the English language) originated in Ancient Egypt. (The Romans influenced, and were influenced, by many cultures.) The Egyptian form of writing is called *"Mdu Ntr," Medu Neter or the hieroglyphics of KMT, which means the Language of the Gods*. The characters, sometimes called ideographs, pictographs or phonograms, are symbols or pictures used to represent sounds or words. From these Ancient Egyptian hieroglyphs, letters were created. Each letter shape can be traced back to a hieroglyph, and the hieroglyph itself (or its meaning) can be directly connected to the way in which we use that letter on a daily basis.

How wonderful it would be for me to regale you with a story about the origin of each of our 26 Roman letters, but that would take a whole book — and that is something for another time. Instead, let's focus on the Roman letters A, B, D, and P, as well as the connection between the Gods and letters "G" and "N." The origins of these letters range from simple to complex, and provide a broad view of how the Roman alphabet came to be.

A IS FOR "APED/VULTURE

It is fairly safe to say that the letter "A" is one of, if not, the first letter children learn. As I mentioned, it is highly likely that a child first learns "A is for apple". What that child doesn't get taught is that "A" stands for lots of other things that actually better relate to the letter itself. After all, an A is a high reaching letter coming to a point; a round apple looks nothing like an A.

In ancient times, for example, a child might have been told "A is for aped." The Egyptian word "aped" is represented by a hieroglyph of a bird; and translates to the scientific word for bird (more specifically, vulture). The vulture ("aped") has a bad reputation these days, but was originally known for being a high-flying bird that valiantly cared for its young. The aped was also considered the Pharaoh's favorite bird. Clearly, the aped had a high station in the culture, making it a great choice for the first letter of the alphabet.

Digging deeper, let's look at the qualities represented by the letter A itself, and how those qualities are related to the aped. The A is reminiscent of pyramids; it is a triangle with great heights. Further, the aped is linked to words like "Air"… "Altitude"… "Ascend" … "Appreciate" — words that all have meanings connected to greatness, height and direction. These words' meanings, coupled with the fact that the letter A is represented by a distinct and greatly appreciated bird, are all indicators of why the capital letter A itself is visually tall and reminiscent of height.

There is a second 'glyph' represented by an arm, thus the word arm. And, for example, it is the "a" in leverage. Thus, one would have to make a distinction between which glyph is represented in the word in question. This will be elaborated further in my book, along with many other examples.

Further, the great Egyptian God Amun, an incredibly influential and powerful God, is later called "Amen," the same word used by many religions to end a prayer. The importance of the A is so great that it is used, in part, to finalize the hopes and thoughts of multitudes of people to ensure that they are heard and responded to by their equivalent of the great Egyptian God Amun. Jumping ahead, Amun is an ascended / high and wise/seeing god.

B IS FOR BARE FOOT

In continuing with our exploration into letter origins, let's look at the letter "B". It originates from the hieroglyph of a bare foot. Among the first qualities we can associate with a bare foot is down (or downward) as the bare foot is at the bottom, or base, of the body. (Can you see a pattern emerging?) The bare foot is support for the body, like a brace or the base of a table. The bare foot helps with movement, bringing you to where you need to be. "Bottom"... "Base"... "Brace"... "Bring"... These words indicate support in both stillness and movement.

The letter B itself is sturdy. The bottom, larger than the top, stabilizes the letter, holding the letter upright, just as the bare foot holds up the rest of the body. When we look at the shape of the lowercase "b," we see its appearance is very similar to that of a leg and barefoot. Other examples of how the letter shows up in our language include: "Boots on the ground" and "Battalion," both representing foot soldiers.

D IS FOR DIGITS /HAND

The letter "D" originated from the hieroglyphic symbol of a hand. The Egyptian word for hand is drrt , The function of the hand (because of our opposable thumbs) separates man from the animals. Man does many things with his hand(s). Among the words that start with D, and are connected to the hieroglyph, is the word "digits," i.e., the fingers of the hand. Digits help man "Do" things… "Duty"… "Drive"… "Diligence." These words are all connected to man doing and accomplishing something. Even more closely linked to the letter D and the hieroglyph of the hand are words such as "dexterous" and "dexterity." The meanings of these words are directly related to hands and the ability of the hand to perform tasks. Thus, D has the quality of action and is directly related to the action of the hand. *Even though the English word hand does not start with the letter d its meaning is consistent in the word.*

▢ P IS FOR PORTAL/DOOR

You may be wondering why I chose to jump all the way to "P" at this point. It's because of the very interesting connection between two letters that I want to share with you. The Egyptian hieroglyph for "P" is a square, more specifically, a door. Now, think about the letter D again. If you were to turn the lowercase letter "d" around (by 180 degrees), what would you have? Yes! A small letter "p"! The d in the picture of the door that we see in the hieroglyph is truly a p, as in the word "Portal." I also looked across languages in Spanish you have puerta.

While it might not be your first thought, when considering doors or portals, we are truly thinking of going out into an open space or a place that affords opportunity (opportunity having the double-p, or two portals… even the word "port" is embedded in "opportunity"). The letter P is instrumental in many common sayings, including, "When opportunity knocks, answer the door" and "window of opportunity." These sayings allude to the double-p (two portals) in opportunity, and the door or portal at which to respond to the opportunity being given to you. So the quality of a door to be considered is that it is an opening, something you can go through. The words that come to mind are: passage...privilege...progress....port....peer (as in look through).

THE LETTERS OF THE GODS

A deeper analysis of letters and hieroglyphs reveals the remarkable way in which some letters correlate with the ancient Gods worshipped by the Egyptians. To appreciate the connection between the two you need to know a bit about Egyptian Cosmology.

Cosmology in general is the study of origins and the universe. Egyptian cosmology revolves around the required balance between humans and the Gods. Humans believed that if they were cooperative, kind and just to one another, the Gods would, in turn, be kind and keep the forces of nature in balance. There are many Gods in Egyptian Cosmology: The God of the ground/earth (Geb), the God of the night/sky (Goddess Nut), the God of the sun (Re), the God of air (Shu) and the God of chaos (Nu). I'm going to focus on the first two Gods, Geb and Nut, for the next part of our journey through the alphabet.

G IS FOR "GEB

The letter "G" comes from the hieroglyphic letter or symbol for the stool. In this respect, the stool is defined as a stand upon which you put a jar. That definition suggests support, foundation, and a most telling word, "grounding" (the stool is on the ground). The "G" also represents the Egyptian God, Geb. As previously mentioned, Geb is the God of earth itself. Egyptian cosmology states that Geb is quite literally the earth ▯ the "ground"... the "geography"... the "globe". The earth "gives" and supports life. The earth "grows; "it generates." As a result, it makes perfect sense for the letter "G" to come out of a symbol that represents an object that grounds and supports, and is the foundation for other objects and beings. Geb is also shown supporting or holding up Nut, the night/sky. Geb is Nut's husband/brother. Does that give you something to consider regarding the ancient wisdom for the need to support?

∧∧∧∧ N IS FOR NUT

The letter "N" originated from the hieroglyph of wavy lines, similar to waves and water. Some say that N represents water, which is a source of life. Also, similar to the letter G, the Roman letter N is connected to both Egyptian hieroglyphs and the Egyptian Gods.

In Egyptian Cosmology, there is the Goddess Nut. She gave birth to the sun, and the sun revolves around her body in a 24-hour cycle to make night and day. Nut is commonly depicted as a woman who is arched over the earth (Geb) on hands and feet. The Goddess Nut is representative of the barrier between chaos and the cosmos and is seen as a protector of the dead whom she keeps with her in her starry sky.

The Goddess Nut is the night, the darkness from which everything derives. In English, she is the "Night". In Spanish, she is the "Noche"... in French "Nuit"... in Greek "Nyx" ... Nacht in German ... "Nox" in Latin ... in Sanskrit

"Naktam" and in Hindi "Nishaa."

"Nyx" (Ancient Greek: Νυξ, "night")" in the Latin translation is the Greek goddess, or personification, of the night. A shadowy figure, Nyx stood at or near the beginning of creation and was the mother of other personified Gods such as Hypnos (Sleep) and Thánatos (Death). Nyx's appearances in mythology are few and far between, but what has been revealed about her is that she is a figure of exceptional power and beauty. Nyx is found in the shadows of the world and is only ever seen in glimpses. As you get away from the source, the object or concept can gain other interpretations.

When we see the reference to Nut as protector of death, it represents that, as time went on, words that were powerful from the opposite quality. The words that come to mind are Engish "no" ... Spanish "nada," ...german "nicht", " nein"

I urge you to continue with your own exploration of the word "night", its spellings and meanings across languages. It is unlikely that the Gods from one belief system to the next can be so similar in both names and existence without it being anything less than purposeful.

So... what does all of this Goddess Nut and Night talk have to do with the Roman letter N? Well, the letter N is derived directly from Nut. And, again, Nut is the night, a bringer of life (like the water depicted in the hieroglyph), and the protector of the dead. Nut's role is natural and nurturing. Nut is the N in origin, beginning, expansive and garden. She is the N in neuter, as she was disempowered through time and forgotten for her role as giving birth to the son. And, what about the word "not" representing further neutralization and negation? As you look at how she is depicted, with her arching body, you can see she is the N in expansive beginning and origin. She is also the N in the words span and extend over or across something, like space and time.

The capital letter N looks physically similar to the waves in the hieroglyph. Interestingly, the depiction of Nut in her arched form is also similar in shape to the lowercase Roman "n". These connections between Roman letters, hieroglyphs, and Ancient Egyptian Gods cannot be ignored or thrown aside. These connections are very much real.

Ok, I Can See It. But Why Should I Care?

While reading thus far, have you said to yourself, "this may be interesting, but how can I use this information?" Or, are you thinking that this chapter satisfies a little curiosity, but that's it; you'll move on to something else because this information does not have any real purpose for you. How can you actually use this in your life?

Doesn't this understanding of letters make them seem so much more alive? Have you not gained a greater appreciation for the letters we use to construct our most meaningful of words? Consider for just a moment how much more enlightening the learning of the Roman alphabet could be to a five-year-old child if he or she were taught by way of hieroglyphics, meaning and origin. The very nature of learning would be greatly enhanced.

Children would not only learn what each hieroglyphic and Roman letter looks like, but would also understand their meanings. Learning the origin of each letter provides the opportunity to more fully grasp the how and why of each shape and sound, as well as the connection of these shapes and sounds to the bigger piece reading words as a whole. Further, understanding each letter's origin enhances the learning of vocabulary and spelling by making connections with the meaning of letters and the purpose each holds within a word. The more we use our five senses to learn, the more mastery we can have. *Children could be encouraged to put letters together to create their own words, another form of creativity and another way to tell their story. I invite you to consider additional uses for this information.*

BUT I'M BEYOND LEARNING TO READ

Pictures provide a very profound way to anchor learning and memory. Further, pictures and words, particularly when they work together, are exceptionally useful tools for drawing you in to a subject. Graphic artists are taught to come up with abstract ideas and create logos to convey meaning, (the same thought process used to create the hieroglyphics) while advertisers use words and pictures to gain access to your mind and influence your perception.

As an example, let's talk about the soda 7UP®. Would the brand name affect you the same way if it were 7b? (The b that is downward and associated with the bare foot.) No, of course it wouldn't, because, in its essence, 7b is a "downer." So, instead, we are sold 7UP, which includes the letter P associated with an upward door, an opening and an *opportunity* for something. The brand name 7UP is pure genius. Without the understanding and purpose of our letters, we are unable to understand the cause and effect of what we are seeing.

Also, by unlocking the meaning of letters, you can cross check the dictionary or encyclopedia and go beyond the history of the words, the etymology to understand how letters and words interact with each other. What are the letters really saying? Why is it that a word can mean something in one language, but mean something completely different in another language? When you explore the reference tools I just mentioned, you see that the meaning of a word changes according to the culture and powers that be at the time. Now you have the tools to see how the story of the letters supports the dictionary meaning, or not, and why.

Learning occurs in stages; since this is an introduction I chose words to represent the concepts presented, primarily having the letter at the beginning of the word. Once there is a command of the concept you begin to see its function in any part of the word.

Further, we can empower children by providing them with an understanding of the meanings and origins of the letters in their names. We can challenge them to personify each letter and gain strength, courage and leadership skills based on the history associated with their names. The big picture impact is that we can teach children to read and write with this new perspective. We can use the origin and meaning of letters to create logos and company names that are more powerful and impactful than ever before. We can provide another efficient way to remember names by seeing what the letters in the name say. We can advance into the future by using the keys provided by our world's ancient history and earliest writing.

If you would like more information about hieroglyphics in general, or want to learn more about the meaning of a specific letter or word, like your name, please feel free to contact me at jahkey2@yahoo.com.

How to Make Your Advertisement Infinitely More Effective

FRANCIS ABLOLA

What we're going to talk about in this chapter is how to focus a laser beam on your target audience when advertising. It's not going to be about writing your sales letter and writing your copy. I'm a direct response copywriter. What that means is I write copy that produces results immediately. But before any single word is written on a page, I want to make sure that I have the audience in mind. How do I do this? Through mind reading. I know it's a little funny to talk about mind reading, but How to Make Your Advertisement Infinitely More Effective is really about getting inside the customer's mind and figuring out exactly what that individual desires. There's a quote I want to share with you. It's by Robert Collier, who's one of the greatest copywriters to ever live. It states, "Always enter the conversation already taking place in the customer's mind."

Now if you're not taking notes right now, you should be. I want you to write this down ... "Always enter the conversation already taking place in the customer's mind." Because as we go through each day, all of us have something that's so pressing in our heads that we need to just get it out into the world. If someone can actually go in there, into our heads, and solve the problem for us, the one that we're thinking about constantly, it immediately cuts through the clutter of everyday thinking and allows them to really reach us. So, that's what we're going to talk about, how you can get into the customer's mind with your marketing.

My promise for everybody reading this is that I'm going to walk you through some powerful influence strategies for increasing the effectiveness of any marketing, of any business or any stage of business. If you're just getting started, you need to know this information; if you've been in business for years, if you're a veteran, and you're not doing this in your business right now, you're leaving money on the table because your advertising is not as effective as it could be.

Did you ever wish that you were a super hero? I think we all might have at some time in our lives. And as a marketer there's one super power that I would want and that's the ability to read people's minds. I would want to get into their heads and actually figure out what they want, even if they, themselves, don't truly know what they want. That's really what we're going to talk about today. It's marketing mind reading.

Now imagine having the power to focus only on attracting your ideal customers, having the ability to build trust instantly with everyone you work with, being able to stay on top of the mind of someone who's looking at your advertising, someone who could be a potential customer of yours, with the power to channel existing wants and desires into your business.

Let's say your business already channels the existing wants and desires of your customers. Can you imagine having the power to press all their emotional hot buttons and psychological triggers so that you send them into a buying frenzy? Wouldn't you like that?

Businesspeople—they have a product, it's their baby. They like to think they know everything that everybody wants, but it's simply not the truth. Yet, that's what we're going to go into today. Imagine having a magical marketing crystal ball that tells you exactly how your ideal customer is thinking and feeling. Now we all can't have that magic ball, but you can use top secret intelligence to create irresistible advertising that fuels your business.

I'm super excited to share that top secret intelligence with you today. When you do these things, you make your ideal customers pay attention. Now, we're so bombarded with information, it's hard to focus on anything. But if you really make your ideal customers pay attention to you, that's a very, very strong thing you can do. They should see you as a trusted advisor and a friend and an authority. Being an authority in your marketplace is a must. Being able to turn that authority into more leads, more loyal customers and eventually more sales, well that's the ultimate super power.

I think everybody reading this wants more sales, so I hope you're with me on that. It really doesn't matter if you're just getting started, if you've been in business for decades or what nature of industry you're in. A lot of people say, "Well, my business is different." Using this strategy, this thing I'm about to show you, every business is the same—because human nature is the same. And that's really what we're planning on using in our advertising.

What I want to show you today is going to help you make an immediate, dramatic impact to your product. But before we go on, I want to answer the question: who the heck is this guy? Some of my early mentors were Les Brown, the legendary Jim Rohn (who was the mentor of Tony Robbins) and William Bailey (who was the mentor Les Brown and Jim Rohn). Today, I'm considered a top marketing and advertising strategist. I work with Fortune 1000 companies, and I've also worked with garage start-ups. Lots of multimillion-dollar CEOs, and New York Times best-selling authors. I've been featured in papers and websites all around the country. I'm also the number-one Amazon best selling author of The Art and Science of Success, with many other best-selling authors. The gurus actually call on me to produce more revenue for their advertising campaigns. This strategy that I'm sharing with you, is going to help you do the same. I've helped my clients create millions in revenue, hundreds of thousands of new leads and customers in rapid speed.

But none of that stuff really matters. What really matters is getting what's inside of my head working for you as if you had a mini me helping grow your business. Let's really get started, because everything we're going to show is actionable, and immediately beneficial to you.

Here's the big problem: we're all overloaded with information. We're overloaded, you're overloaded, your prospects and your customers are overloaded. It's been said that we are bombarded with some 3000 advertisements per day. How do we get our prospect's attention? That's really what we're fighting for with everything going on in the world today. The first solution that everyone goes to is advertise. But how do we know we're doing the right thing? There are so many things we can do ... TV, radio, internet, social media, press releases and online classified ads. There are so many different channels as a marketer, and as an advertiser, that we can use. But how do we know it's effective? How do we know we're using our time the right way? How do we know we're using our money the right way? As an entrepreneur, I'm sure you'd agree that money and time are the two most important things in a business.

So really what we want to do is focus in on effective advertising. And here's what effective advertising does … Effective advertising focuses on the right media to the right potential customer. If your advertising doesn't do that, if it goes to a broad audience, you may be losing money. Does your advertisement speak directly to your target audience? Effective advertising speaks to the person who's reading it. Not only that, but it is benefit driven to what your ideal customer wants. Not what the marketer wants but what they're customer is looking for. And finally, it has a specific call-to-action. If you're advertising doesn't do this, you may be leaving money on the table.

As an example, you wouldn't stick a realtor sign up on the front lawn of a home to attract a million-dollar buyer, would you? Really, it's comparing your advertising to a shotgun, versus a sniper rifle. All of your advertising should be the sniper rifle, especially if you have a small budget to work with.

Here's the bad news: all of your customers are ignoring you. You really need to cut through the clutter. You need to get their attention with laser focus and that sniper rifle approach. So, who do your customers listen to? I've eluded to this earlier, they listen to trusted friends and advisors. They listen to people who understand their needs, their problems and have their best interest in mind. David Ogilvy, one of my legendary heroes in marketing, wrote, "All good marketing requires empathy." It's very important, it's another writer-downer, if you're taking notes. "All good marketing requires empathy." That means having a connection with your target audience but calling them a person, because that's what they really are.

So how do you reach all these real people? Too many business owners tend to get their advertising and their marketing done the wrong way. One of the ways they get marketing done wrong is they try to sell the features and not the benefits of what someone is looking for. They market to what they think is important verses what the customer's looking for. They don't think what the customer thinks is important.

Now, there may be some people out there thinking, "Well, that's not me. I didn't do this when I started my marketing campaigns, and we're making a lot of good money right now." But the fact is, it doesn't matter if you're losing money or making money, if you don't know your customer market—even if you're doing well with your marketing—chances are you can probably increase your sales and conversions. It doesn't always mean you're going to fail by not using this approach first, but it almost always means you're going to increase conversions by going back and doing this kind of research.

Here's what I want to stress today. You can be a terrible advertisement copywriter, but as long as you know your market with pinpoint accuracy, you can create effective advertising. My advice might seem counter-intuitive … and that's to stop selling to customers. Instead, you want to listen to your customers, and you want to become their best friends, their BFFs. The reason why is because you want to position yourself as a trusted advisor offering valuable guidance to your best friend. That puts you in a completely different category from all the people who aren't listening to your market but are just trying to sell to them.

When you become a trusted advisor, you become the first person this customer listens to. You become their expert and their authority. You become your target market--thinking what they think, feeling what they feel, going where they go, and experiencing what they experience.

Now, I became a really good copywriter in my niche, but not because I'm a great writer. In fact, I barely made it out of college English. I barely made it out of high school. The reason I became a really good copywriter in my niche is because I understand what my audience is looking for. I actually go to seminars as an attendee to talk with the people who are there, to do my market research, to get into their heads, to feel what they feel and to experience what they experience.

If you're selling to a market, and it's your primary market, you want to become that market, not a person selling to them. This is so vitally important. Stop thinking customer, prospect, or name on a list. Start thinking "real person" with hopes, dreams, wants, needs, desires, and problems only you can solve.

I have a funny approach to doing this that I call making up "imaginary best friends" for fun and profit. Because I love my best friends. And becoming someone's best friend is the next best thing to climbing into their head and reading their mind. Again, going back to the super powers that we all wish we had, mine is being able to read somebody's mind. If you can't read somebody's mind, the next best thing is becoming best friends with them, because best friends tell each other secrets. They tell each other hopes and dreams and desires. They let you know what they want, why they want it, what they like, who they trust, why they trust them, and why they buy.

If I consider you a really good friend, we share things that we wouldn't share to the general public. And I'm sure people reading this today have the same thing with their best friend. So, I want you to imagine being best friends with your marketplace. And here's the thing, your imaginary best friends? What we do is call it creating customer personas, or often times creating customer avatars. Basically, it's a clear, written profile of specific segments of your target audience.

When you have this, you can actually identify to the "T" who the person your ideal customer is. You want to focus on attracting who will give you the most money with the least resistance. This may seem like I'm saying you should get more for doing less. But it's not; it's about making the most money with the least amount of resistance.

Zero in on your best customers. Zero in on the people who you enjoy working with, and who also enjoy working with you. Think about it ... Would you rather work with the guy who enjoys going golfing a couple of afternoons per week, or another guy, the party animal? The answer really depends on what you want and what you have to offer. But the marketing is different, the advertising is different, to go after these two different groups of people. When you're creating imaginary friends, it really helps to interact with your target customer on a deeper, individual basis. After all, what you're doing here is building a lifestyle business.

You always want to think in terms of what benefits they want, not what you can offer them; not what you think they want, but what they're actually looking for. You must remember this for when you get into the marketplace, for when you create these imaginary friends, for when you truly begin to understand what they're looking for, because you might come to find out they're looking for something completely different than what you have to offer and that they're only working with you because that's the closest thing. This is exciting, because you now have the opportunity to get more money or work from them by creating a different relationship—all because they're looking for something that's not on the market. Who knows? This could even be a new opportunity for you and your business.

Creating imaginary friends also guides your marketing: it guides your brand, it guides design, and it guides advertising messages that speak to the proper audience. Again, we're seeing the shotgun versus the sniper rifle approach. So let's make some imaginary friends. I'm about to walk you through a process that I use whenever I create a marketing piece for a new audience, or a new market.

I'd like to say I'm not alone, because I have my imaginary friends who are helping me write my marketing. Again, this is the guide to effective advertising, even before writing a single word on a page, or creating a single ad. It's creating these imaginary friends, who tell you exactly what your market's looking for.

STEP 1

The first step is to brainstorm. It's sitting down with a pad and paper and just thinking. "Who are your best customers? Who are they currently? What type of customers do you want to attract? Who would you consider a best customer for you?" When you create these imaginary friends, think of them as they fit into each segment of your customer base. You don't need only one imaginary best friend, you can have multiple imaginary friends who all speak to a different audience.

You want to give them names and personalities, even jobs and families. Be very specific with the information you already know. If you already have customers, you can say, "Well, this is Bob. Bob works full-time, but he also works on the side as a real estate investor. He's looking to be more effective. You know, Bob works 40 hours a week in his regular job, and he spends about 20 hours a week in his real estate investing business. He also has a family and two kids that he tries to juggle with, and he's very frustrated with the results he's getting in this side business."

Knowing all this information, you get to know Bob a little bit better, and how to help him even more. So far this is really just an educated guess, because the next thing you want to do is actually go out in market and prove it. You want to go gather the data. You want to see, do these people really exist? The best way to do that is to actually go and look to your existing customers, go and talk to them. Talk to anybody in your company who interacts with your customers on a daily basis. If you have sales people in your company, for example, talk to them. Maybe talk to them about their best customers.

If you have a best customer in mind, talk to them, ask them what they want. Start doing interviews. The best thing you can do, the easiest thing, is you can survey your list by using a tool like SurveyMonkey or Wufoo. These let you create free forms to send out via email, asking your list of "friends" questions that will help you get to know them better. And by getting to know them better, your advertising becomes much more effective, because you gear all of your marketing message directly to these friends. This is actually how I won the award for copywriter of the year and became the guru's go-to guy. In my market I write heavily to people who want to learn how to become real estate investors. So I go where they go, and I get to know them. I actually go to seminars and sit in the back of the room. I talk to people who are attending—just like I was the seminar for the first time.

I get to know them better, and I find ways to understand them better, to feel what they feel, to understand their emotions, to experience the experiences they go through. And by doing that you discover so many things about your target market that you'll never know just from graphs and data and not seeing customers face-to-face. It's super important to do this, to get to know them and become friends with them. Open up a conversation (and it's amazing to know what kinds of information people give just by opening up a conversation).

STEP 2

The next step is to dig deeper. From the information you've gathered, from the brainstorming you've done and from all the proof you've backed it up with, you want to ... understand who they are, what they want, how they buy, why they buy, and what would get them to buy from you? Obviously, this is a very important question.

STEP 3

Now is the time to create your customer profile. That's right: create a profile of your imaginary friends, and make them as real as possible. I even go to the extent of finding a picture that best represents the person. I actually go to Google images or use a service like iStockphoto or Dreamstime. If you know your target market is male, in his 40s or 50s, with a family, you can actually go to istockphoto.com and find photos of people just like that.

By having these profiles and by getting them as real as possible, you can create this avatar, this persona, this imaginary friend who you can speak to and write to. Just the other day, we were talking to one of my copywriter friends on an interview we did, and he was referencing another copywriter who's a very successful copywriter. On her first promotion she was writing to a market her mother actually fit into. So as her customer avatar, as her persona, and as her imaginary friend, she actually set a picture of her mom in front of her laptop, and as she wrote the letter and the advertising piece, she wrote it as if she was writing to her mother. The advertisement piece was a well-liked hit, and it was very, very successful. Imagine you're writing your advertising to someone you truly care about, who you truly want to see a difference in. This is when and why your advertising becomes so much more powerful.

Here's what you want to ask when you're really digging into creating these imaginary friends. The first one is demographics, it's the who they are. Let's say this is Bob. What do we want to know about Bob? We want to know where he lives, his age group, marital status, occupation, job status and income. Does he own a home, does he rent? What's his education and reading level? That's really important, especially when you're creating an advertisement. What kind of lifestyle does he live? What kind of things interest him? What are his special interests? Maybe it's political interest, something like that. And political affiliations are very important to know, because obviously political affiliations really drive a person's character and how they operate. For example, you don't want to write a message that has a Democrat overtone to a Republican audience. It doesn't work that way.

STEP 4

The next thing is psychographics. This is about what they want and how they see themselves. What's their personal attitude toward themselves? Are they confident or are they not confident about their future? How do you use that in your advertising? How do they interact with you and other people? What are their personality types? Are they outgoing or are they soft-spoken? It's really important to know how to approach a target audience through their certain mannerisms. What are their beliefs? Again, really important. You want to make sure that you're not offending your target audience, but you also don't want to go too soft and make them ignore your advertising. What kind of affiliations in other groups do they have? What's their social status? Where do they see themselves in the world, and how the world reacts to them? What kind of books do they enjoy reading? This is really important. You're getting back into the conversation that's going in their head. If you know they're a huge Twilight fan (Twilight was a huge book on the market), you could actually use Twilight in your advertisement—maybe as a subject line? What websites have they visited? Also note that they're diehard Huffington Post readers. Why? If you've created an advertisement that actually talked about the Huffington Post it would attract them and actually get them to open the advertisement. What kind of hobbies do they do? Again, if they have strong beliefs in a certain hobby, how do you use that in your marketing? And what drives them on a day-to-day basis? Note: All these questions are important, but I think more important than the demographic information, is what they want and how they interact with you.

I also want to add a quick word about websites. I love forums. I love forums because people go to forums to talk with somebody in the same exact niche. It's two people having a conversation who are friends. Everybody chimes in, so you get to know your market well. Dashboards.com is a great website for finding niche forums like that. People open up and act like themselves inside of forums because they're not buying stuff. They feel like they can talk like they would normally talk to their friends. A point to add to the forums is that when people interact on forums, they're actually hidden by their usernames. They can even share their deepest feelings. This goes back to getting into where your market goes. It's not even real life, person-to-person, but it's going to allow you to see them where they spend time and interact with others. Very important, I love this strategy.

Going back to the point of what drives them on a day-to-day basis, what do they focus on? Are they focusing on just surviving a daily life? Or are they looking to connect with others? Are they looking for affluence and significance in their family life? Are they looking for enjoyment on a daily basis? When you understand the true psychological need, what they need to fulfill, your advertising becomes much more effective.

STEP 5

Find the pain. What's really eating away at them, day and night? What's the primary need your imaginary friend is desperate to fill? What's the biggest problem that's always on their mind? What keeps them up at night? Get into the conversation that's already happening on an everyday basis. What problems are they trying to solve in their lives? What's the biggest benefit they want? When you start thinking of what needs they are desperate to fill, and approaching your marketing that way, it becomes so much more effective because it clears the clutter. It stops you from saying "Here's what I think is important to you," but, rather, allows you to say, "This is what seems to be important from your point of view." You begin to be able to understand what influences their decisions. Again, this is a very important part of understanding who your customer is and what is their ultimate goal in buying from or interacting with you. Why are they looking to buy this product or service, if they don't know that they want to buy this product or service? What needs are they looking to fill that will get them to respond to your advertising? What emotions do you want them to feel? Is it security, is it confidence? Do you want them to feel significant when they work with you or buy your product or service? Do you want to give them independence? Are they looking for independence when they buy or interact with you? Also is it fun for them? What would make it fun to work with you? Again, a very important thing to know. Do they trust you? Hopefully the message that has woven its way throughout this entire presentation will lead you to understand that the whole point is getting your customers to trust you as an advisor they can call upon and lean on. And finally, if they don't trust you yet, what has to happen for them to trust you? What are they looking for as a symbol of trust?

A good example of that last point is your mailbox. How many things do you get in the mail for free? People who are sending you free gifts are putting you in a "wow" state of mind, like, "This guy's great. He just gave me something free." It automatically breaks down barriers. But it's also building value upfront, so you have their trust later. This is very, very important. How do you stand out? How do you create that "wow" experience? How are you different? And how do you create that trust to carry you into a deeper relationship. When you're creating that trust, you want to create your trust with your ideal client, which takes us into what we we're going to talk about now, which is how do you focus only on your imaginary friend, who you can help and, more importantly, who wants your help? You can't help everyone, especially if they don't want to hear from you.

So how do you only work with those people who are actively looking for what you have to offer? How do you invest your time and energy on clients and customers who can help expand your business and move in the direction that you want? The answer? You only focus on working with clients and consumers who want that same thing you are offering and who will also support your lifestyle in terms of that.

You also want to avoid time wasters. Don't work with energy vampires, because these people will take your business away from you. Only focus on the imaginary friends, the customer group that most wants your help, and that you can help the most by giving them massive transformational value.

STEP 6

Put your imaginary friends to work. Now that you've created all these profiles, that you've put these pieces together, how do you put them to work?

The simplest thing is, think of your new imaginary friend every time you plan a new campaign, or craft, or sales message. Again, all of your advertising is driven (laser-focused) to that specific person. So as you're creating your marketing, as you're creating your websites and as you're creating your copy, think of, "Does my imaginary friend, or will my imaginary friend, respond to this piece of advertising?"

The next thing is to speak to that individual. Here's a trick: all of your advertisements should speak to an individual person, not a group. Because when we read advertisements, we don't feel like we're a group, we feel like we're a single person, because we really are. And your advertisements should portray that. Develop a relationship with your imaginary friend. The more you get to know your imaginary friends, the more you get to know your marketplace. The more you get to know your marketplace, the easier it is to speak to them through all of the advertisements you put out.

HERE ARE MY BIGGEST TAKEAWAYS

One, become your audience. Watch what they watch, read what they read, go where they go. Two, get into the mind of your ideal prospect. Enter the conversation. Three, focus your advertising on your market. Focus the benefit-driven message that your customer wants. Not you but what your customer wants. Four, the biggest takeaway is talk to your imaginary friend—because best friends share secrets.

I think that's all I've got. I hope you were taking notes, because the most important part of your business is finding out what your customers actually want. It doesn't matter whether you're doing terrible in your marketing efforts or if you think you're doing well, applying these techniques will skyrocket your conversions.

Have More Money, More Clients and More Freedom by Going Digital

ASHAR ALAM

As a savvy business owner, you understand that, whatever field you are in, whether it is chiropractic or real estate or Italian food, you are also in the business of marketing. You also know that the key to building and maintaining a successful business lies in keeping your marketing current and effective.

Many traditional forms of marketing simply don't measure up to the digital resources available today. If you haven't embraced this medium yet, you probably have seen competitors who do have a solid digital marketing strategy surging ahead of the pack (that includes you). If your market doesn't have a digital player yet, you have a golden opportunity to leave your competitors behind.

There are several steps you need to take to bring your business digitally up to par, and to get in position to set yourself apart. This chapter of The Authorities will focus on one very powerful digital marketing tool, search engine optimization (usually referred to as SEO). But, first, here's a broad look at exactly what digital marketing is.

DIGITAL MARKETING AUDIT

There are several different questions you should ask yourself in order to assess the current state of your business with respect to digital marketing. The most basic of these is: Do I have a website? If the answer is no, then you need to get one! This is as basic as it gets, but also as essential as it gets. A business's website is really the source from which all other digital marketing strategies flow.

If you do already have a business website, you can pat yourself on the back, but you are not out of the woods yet, not by a long shot. Begin to take a look at how well your site is serving your business:

- **Look critically at your site's URL/domain name.** A domain name like LocksmithSanDiego.com will have a leg up on competitors because it aligns well with what prospects for that business would be searching for on the web. It's also important to realize that a ".com" — or country-specific domains like ".ca" and ".co.uk" — is generally favored most by search engines and looked at as most legitimate by prospects.

- **Think about keywords that are relevant to your business from a customer's perspective.** Consider your own habits. What would you type into a search engine if you were looking for service in your field? The better optimized for these keywords your site is, the easier it will be for your prospects to find it.

- **Do some research to determine where your site ranks on popular search engines.** There is software that will do this, but it is simpler to do a Google search using likely keywords for your business. Does your site come up in the first page of results? The second? Again, think about how you use Google. How often do you navigate past the first or second page of search results? Most Googlers won't get too far past the first several results on the first page which, of course, is where you want your site to be. Optimized SEO can help make that happen.

- **How well does your site work when your prospects actually get there?** Can customers buy your product(s) directly from your website? If so, do they buy from you when they visit your website? How much time do they spend on your site once they get there? You can monitor these statistics, as well as other important website performance factors, with resources like Google Analytics; doing so is essential to getting the most out of your website.

- **Do you take advantage of other digital media channels**, such as social media (Facebook, Twitter, etc.), large retailers (Amazon, iTunes, etc.), mobile apps, and SMS marketing?

These questions and considerations represent a good starting point for assessing your business's digital marketing prowess, but they are really just scratching the surface. There are many more things to look into, whether it's calculating return on investment by estimating the lifetime value of your clients, setting up an infrastructure for capturing clients' email addresses and phone numbers, or optimizing your website for mobile devices.

It might seem like a lot to think about, and it is, but the more you apply these principles to your marketing strategy, the more your business will benefit. Everyone knows that putting in the effort is necessary to bringing about the desired result; what the above guidelines do is help you channel that effort strategically and productively.

SEO

Speaking of using your effort wisely, one of the most important aspects of digital marketing is SEO. You will definitely want to funnel some of your digital marketing efforts into SEO to ensure that your prospects have the opportunity to find out about your business.

The name "search engine optimization" is fairly self-explanatory — it refers to optimizing a website so that it's easy for a search engine to find it. However, properly executing this concept is not as simple as the concept itself is. Keywords, like the ones discussed above, must be well-integrated into the very coding of the various pages on your site. There are also several other factors, such as back links, social markers and likability — discussed in further detail below — that contribute to how your site will fare on the search engines.

Crucially, all of this must be done in a strategic way. Obviously catering to keywords can lead to negative repercussions. Search engines will take action against those who blatantly game the system, banishing them to obscure sections of search results and dealing a severe blow to their digital marketing schemes.

"FREE" ADVERTISING

In the sense that it requires time and effort, and potentially the paid help of a specialist, SEO is not free. However, compared to the level of paid advertising you would have to employ to get the same level of visibility, SEO is a terrific bargain. And, it generates a very strong return on investment (ROI).

In terms of search engines, organic SEO can actually be much more valuable than paid advertising, even without considering cost. The major search engines — Google, Yahoo! and Bing — display unpaid listings on the same results page as paid ones. Plus, local business results are typically included with national ones. Most of the time, web users simply ignore the paid listings, which display on a different part of the page —either off to the side or above the organic listings. (Again, think about your own behavior in such situations — you may have never even noticed that Google displays paid listings alongside the unpaid ones you naturally look for.)

People rely on search engines to provide something like an unbiased survey of what's out there, and paid ads don't fit very well into this expectation. On the other hand, a "real" listing that pops up prominently in the results is more appealing. Websites that pop up toward the beginning of the results do so because they are well optimized for search engines. This is the key to SEO. The effort required is invisible to the customer, and a prominent search engine result comes with built-in legitimacy.

WHAT ARE SEARCH RESULTS BASED ON?

You've already seen how SEO starts with keywords. Your search engine ranking will partly be dependent upon where these keywords show up on your site and how much competition there is for the keywords you target. As a general guideline, strategically placed keywords should not exceed 1-2% of the copy on your site.

"Longtail" keywords, such as "best DUI attorney in Buffalo New York," can help sites succeed in a competitive market, although incorporating them will probably require outside help; for example, from a specialty marketing firm. Because SEO is so important these days, many firms specialize in assisting companies in this way. This is, of course, an extra expense — as discussed above, good SEO is not free — but for many markets its benefits will hugely outweigh the costs.

A more stripped down way to achieve something similar is to incorporate a blog into your website. Blogs continually generate fresh, keyword-rich content, and can help drive traffic to your website. For many businesses, generating blog posts is a more doable in-house operation for enhancing SEO, although it is also something that can be outsourced, and typically for a much lower price than that of hiring a marketing firm.

There are other specific attributes besides keywords that are important as well. Some of these are still intimately related to keywords, while others are completely separate. Google will determine rankings according to:

Authority – How authoritative is a given site in relation to the search term? Has it been highly ranked in the results of this search term for a long time?

Relevance – How popular is this search? Is it generating a lot of web traffic? Are many people searching for these specific keywords?

Competition – What sites mention these keywords? What sites prominently feature these keywords (i.e., in the title or domain name)? What are the SEO-related qualities, both on-page and off-page, of these sites? For example, age, rank, back links (see next bullet point), and prominence and density of keywords.

Back links – These are like citations in an article, and function somewhat as votes for a site. How many other sites are linking back to a given page? Are the sites that are linking to the page in question themselves high-SEO sites? Poor quality back links can be worse than no links at all, as this is exactly the type of thing Google cracks down on. Spammy back links can cause a site to be thrown into the Google "sandbox," meaning it is dropped from the top hundred search results.

Social markers – Does this site have connections with social media sites like Facebook, Twitter and LinkedIn? Are users linking back to it on these platforms?

Likability – Many different measures determine the likability of a site, such as:

- Time spent on page – How long do visitors to a given page stay there before navigating away? Videos are a great way to increase visitors' time spent on your site. A live chat feature is another way to keep visitors from navigating away from a page.

- Bounce rate – The percentage of visitors who leave the site rather than navigate to other pages within the site. A high bounce rate means people who visit your site are not finding a reason to stay there.

- Scroll rate – Do visitors scroll down through a page, or leave directly after it loads without scrolling through? Make sure each page has enough content to engage a visitor. Most pages should have a minimum of 500 words. Meeting that word limit is one easy way to address this issue.

- Grammar – Poor grammar can be a marker of regurgitated content. Sites with high likability will not have grammatical errors.

- Downloads – A great way to increase likability of a page. Offering PDF documents, MP3s, and/or video files as downloads helps to engage visitors to your site.

SEO is certainly a multi-layered topic, and the larger world of digital marketing is even more intensive. This chapter has given you several simple action steps you should take immediately to better market your business online. To learn more about how digital marketing can build your business significantly, you may want to visit thebookondigitalmarketing.com.

In the meantime, look back through the audit above, and through the bulleted list of SEO principles. Satisfactorily dealing with these various aspects of digital marketing is often an ongoing project for successful businesses. There are many angles from which to approach it, which means finding a place to dive in is easy — there are so many options.

SEO in particular is a long term consideration. Working your way into a favorable spot in search engine rankings can take time. But, as discussed above, truly earning a prominent organic listing is highly valuable exposure for a business, so it's a worthy goal to pursue.

And, now that you have some valuable information about how to go about it, go out and spread the word about your business!

www.ingramcontent.com/pod-product-compliance
Lightning Source LLC
Chambersburg PA
CBHW050215230526
45470CB00001B/395